THE ART OF
MEHNDI

SUMITA BATRA

CARLTON
BOOKS

THIS IS A CARLTON BOOK

Published in 2013 by Carlton Books Limited
20 Mortimer Street
London W1T 3JW

10 9 8 7 6 5 4 3 2 1

Design and Text © Carlton Books 1999 and 2013

A CIP catalogue for this book is available from the British Library

ISBN 978-1-78097-301-2 (paperback)
ISBN 978-1-78097-321-0 (hardback)

Printed and bound in Dubai

CONTENTS

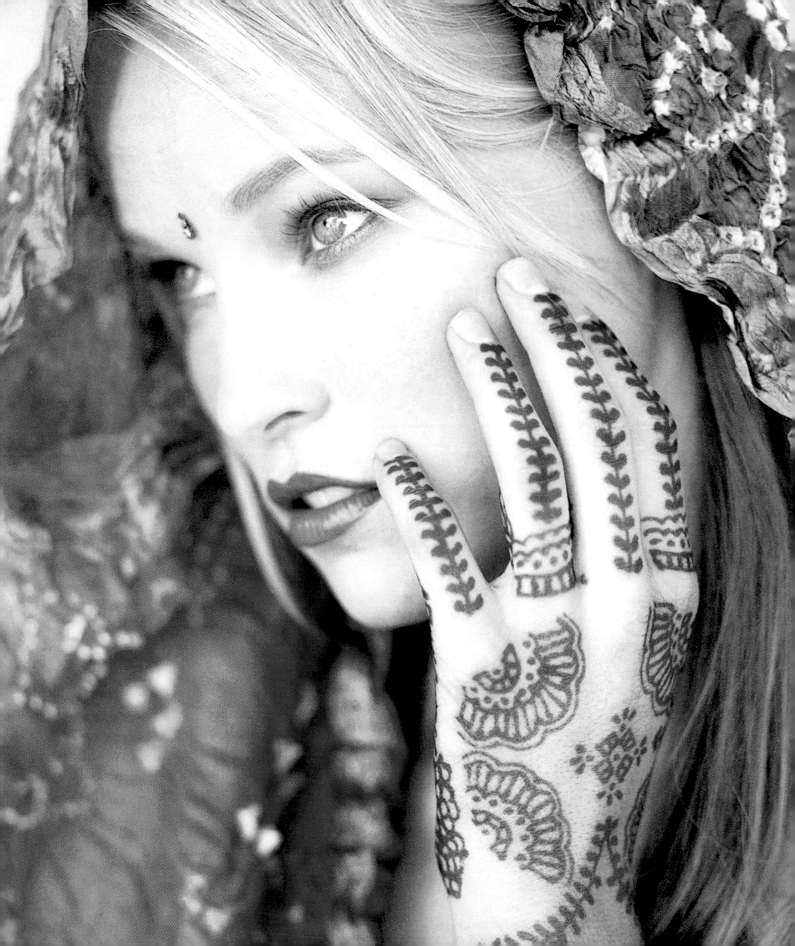

INTRODUCTION

A friend gave me a glass ball, filled halfway with sand and shells. The sand signified time gone by and the shells represented the beautiful things that are left behind. The art of mehndi is one such shell that the sand of time has left behind. It sparkles and perseveres. To the West, it is a temporary tattoo. To the East, it is about women, celebration, hope, transition, growth, auspiciousness, spirituality, good fortune, adornment and, above all, pure beauty.

Mehndi has been around for centuries and crossed all barriers of caste, religion and distance. I believe mehndi brings its own good fortune to the wearer. To me, it has brought tremendous good luck. If I had been told, a few of years ago, that I would be where I am today, I wouldn't have believed it.

I always tell my clients that I paint with the open-hand philosophy – the belief that the surface area of your palm is bigger than that of your fist. If you try to hold something in your fist, you will crush it or reduce its chances for growth. But if you keep your palm open, you will have, give and receive more.

Mehndi belongs to no single caste, culture or country. It is unique, and will bring only beauty into your life. I hope this book gives you a little insight into this beautiful art form.

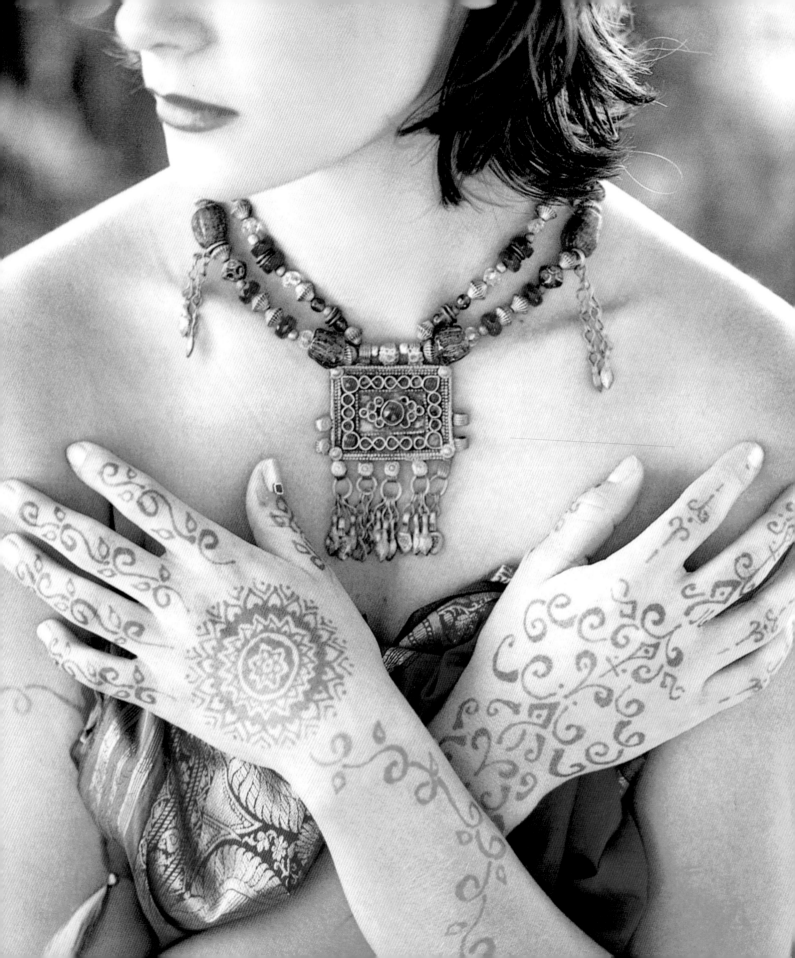

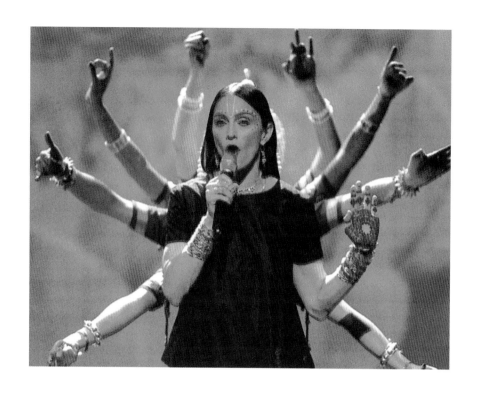

' When Sumita hennas my hands
and feet, I am transported to
another time and place. A world
of magic, passion and romance. '

MADONNA

Henna paste, made from the crushed leaves of the henna plant, was used to colour the skin as long as five thousand years ago. In India, North Africa, South-East Asia and the Middle East, henna is seen as a blessing with the power to bring the wearer happiness and wealth. In the twelfth century, the Moguls are thought to have introduced the art of mehndi to India, where it has long played a significant part in the wedding ritual.

Henna painting spans many countries and religions, but the design details vary from culture to culture. Generally, Indian designs are made up of finely drawn floral and paisley patterns, Arabic designs concentrate on larger floral motifs on the hands and feet, and African designs include bold geometric shapes.

The **art of mehndi** is synonymous with women, who apply henna decoratively to their bodies with intricate designs that have been faithfully passed down from one generation to the next. But because the art of mehndi belongs in a female domain, the chroniclers of history, who were exclusively male, have written little about this absorbing ancient practice.

Chapter 1

HISTORY AND DESIGN SYMBOLISM

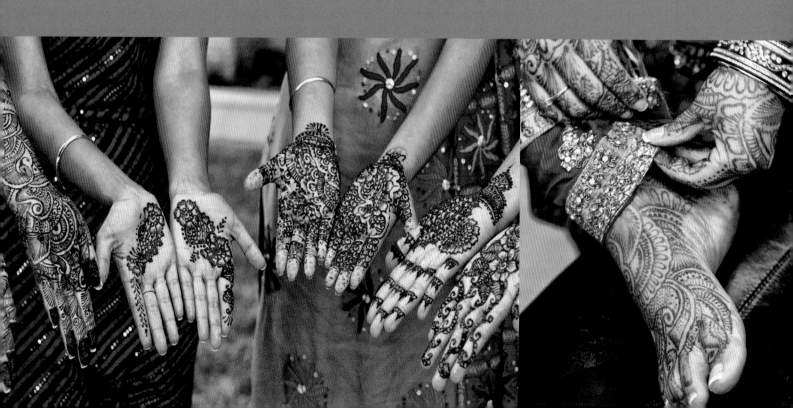

INDIA

*M*ehndi is the Indian word for henna, and mehndi body painting represents a spiritual and therapeutic experience, which is one of the reasons why it is never carried out in haste. After the Moguls brought the art of mehndi from the Middle East in the twelfth century, it soon spread throughout India and Bangladesh.

Most mehndi designs are linked to religious beliefs and practices. For example, a person from Islam prays with their arms open wide and their palms facing skyward. So as not to distract from the prayer, their hands can only be decorated with abstract designs, such as floral motifs. More conspicuous drawings, such as birds and faces, are not allowed.

In India, only the body parts above the navel are considered holy, so any religious symbols, such as a cross or swastika (the sign for purity), must be painted above it. Dancers wear mehndi on the palms of their hands so that the audience can see their movements from a distance, which helps enhance their performance.

WEDDING CUSTOMS

One of the most important occasions for which mehndi is used is the wedding ceremony. Painting the bride's body with henna – the *mehndi raat* (meaning mehndi night) – is an essential part of the preparations. It is a ceremony in itself, which has remained unchanged for many years.

It is customary for the bridegroom to supply the bride and other female members of the family with henna. Much is made of its arrival. Usually, the mothers of both the bride and groom dab a little henna into the palms of their soon-to-be-married son and daughter before the serious business of designing begins. Then follows the perfect opportunity for the female members of both families to get to know each other, as they take their time applying the henna amid much teasing and storytelling.

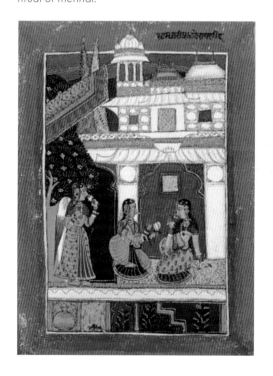

Indian miniature from c. 1690, illustrating the ritual of mehndi.

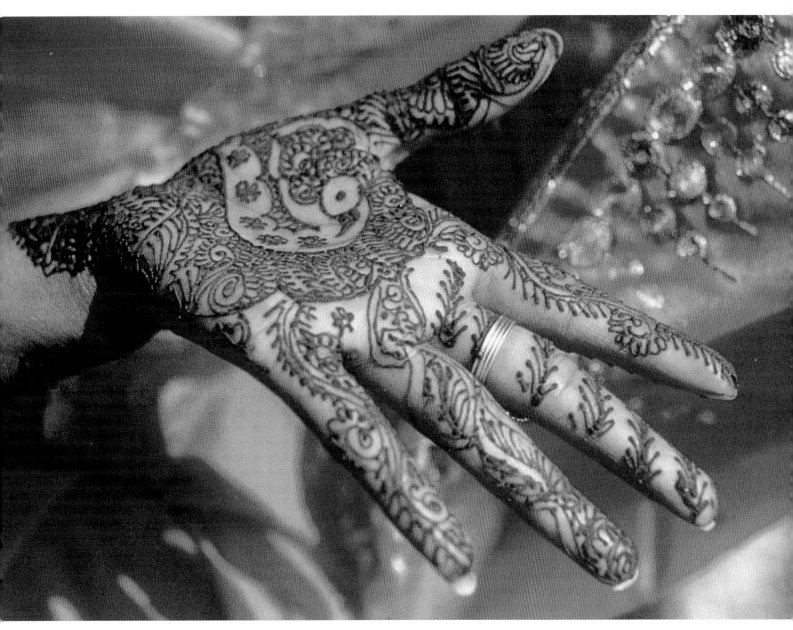

The distinctive paisley shape in the centre of the palm stems from the mango, an aphrodisiac and symbol of passion.

Mehndi is painted on the hands and feet at weddings in almost every religion practiced in India.

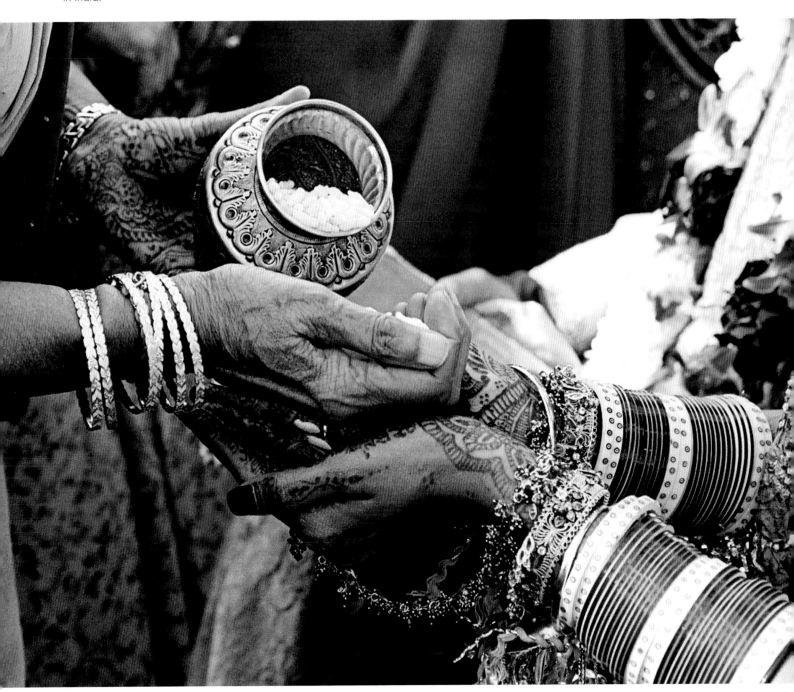

The most popular tale about mehndi traditions claims that the bride-to-be will not have to touch any housework for as long as her henna designs last. During the first month of marriage, a maid will take care of all her household duties, including bathing, so that the new bride will not need to use her hands at all. This allows her plenty of free time to get to know the members of her new family.

Another story tells that the darker the henna stains the skin, the more the groom's mother will love her new daughter-in-law. Because the bride goes to live with her husband's family immediately after the wedding, this is an important consideration. This story is not as far-fetched as it sounds when you consider that originally henna was painstakingly applied with fine toothpick-like sticks. The process could take as long as 24 hours and would require considerable patience from the bride. It follows that the most patient of brides would receive the most intricate decorations and the very deepest stains, proving that she was either naturally endowed with the gift of patience or was willing to learn patience – either way, it was considered a good indication of how well she would get along with others. Even today, in many villages, it is the mother-in-law with whom the bride spends most of her time before the wedding, so it is vital that their relationship is harmonious.

Another popular custom is to hide the initials of the husband-to-be in the mehndi design. On the wedding night, the bride asks her new husband to find the initials. If he is successful, it means that he will be the dominant partner in the marriage, but if he fails, the wife will be the one to rule the relationship. Naturally, the female mehndi artists go to great lengths to conceal the initials in their intricate designs.

These wedding preparations are an enjoyable time for the women, whose job it is to soothe the bride's nerves, and can last for weeks, sometimes months. At times, a bride may be required to remain stock still for as long as 10 hours if the design is particularly complex. Indian weddings celebrated in the West, however, are usually restricted to a tighter time scale and last only a matter of days.

In some sects, especially in Punjab, the groom coats his hand with henna and leaves its imprint on the wall of his house as a reminder of the special event and a symbol of him becoming a man. Many families preserve this for as long as possible.

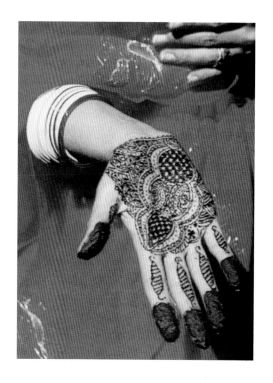

An Indian bride has her hands painted as dark as possible with henna, believing that the deeper the stain, the more her mother-in-law will love her.

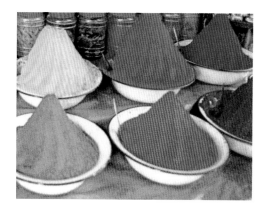

Henna dyes in India are sold in an array of dazzling jewel-bright colours.

Although mehndi decorations fade from black to light brown with everyday wear and washing, they still retain their original beauty (right).

A young bride enjoys the relaxing effect of having her palm decorated the modern way, using a mehndi cone (below).

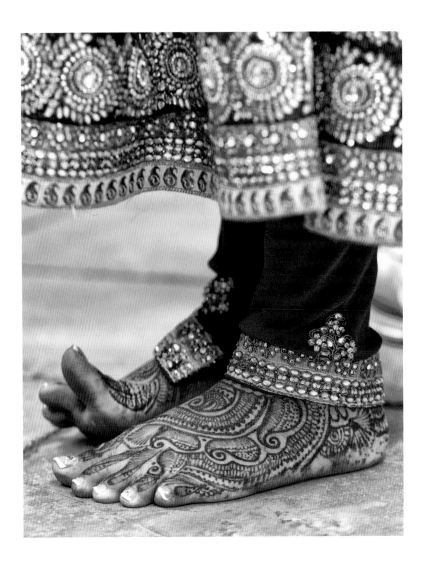

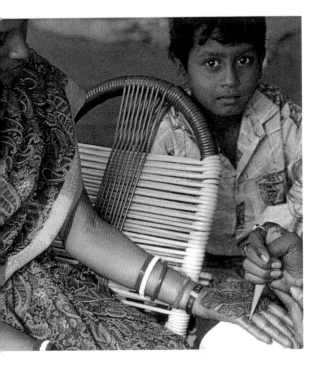

Henna's associations with joy and celebration are regarded as so sacred that a widow must not touch henna because she is no longer supposed to feel joy. Her association with happiness is cut off for good, as she is excluded from all social functions. It is even considered bad luck for her and a bride to look at each other.

As well as her wedding, there are many other significant events and special occasions that occur throughout a woman's life that are either considered a new beginning or a time to celebrate. These include the prayer (*pooia*) before the birth of a child and ceremonies such as *Karwa Chouth*, where women from the Hindu faith pray for the health and long

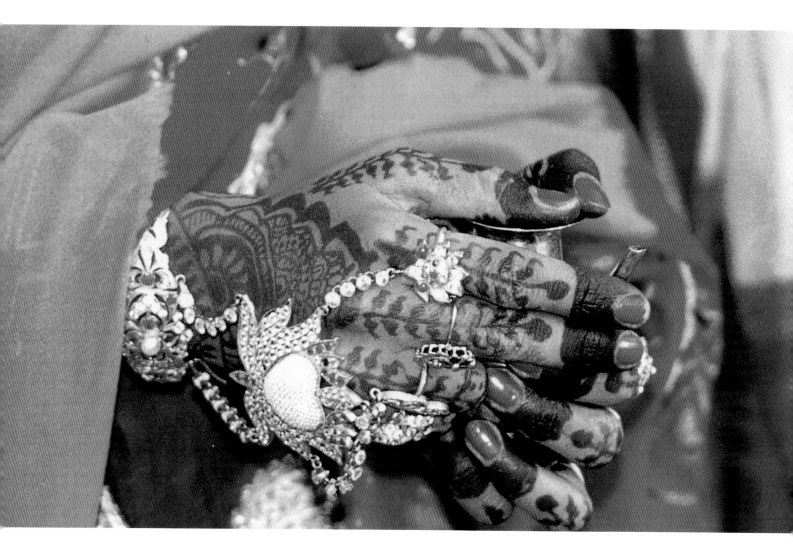

life of their husbands. All these special occasions are celebrated by painting the woman's hands and feet with intricate henna designs.

THE MEANING OF COLOUR

In addition to mehndi, Indian women use colour in their make-up and on their hair to denote social status or religious beliefs. All colours have a symbolic meaning: red is fire, orange represents the rising sun, ochre is blood and pink signifies the earth. Many women dye their partings bright red to indicate they are married, and brides' faces are

Glittering gold jewellery and brightly painted red nails make a striking contrast with the deeply stained hands of a Bombay bride.

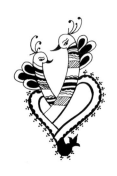

Pair of peacocks

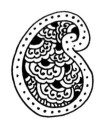

Paisley

Abstract design

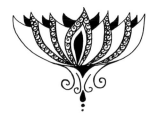

Lotus

beautifully made up with red and white. Mothers put lampblack (*surma*) around their babies' eyes to protect them from the evil eye, and highly religious women paint a marking on their forehead to show their devotion to their god.

In southern and eastern India, the high rainfall means henna is not able to grow. Instead, in the east, they use a red ink called *alta* to sketch simple designs. The practice is completely different in the south where they make a yellow-brown paste from the bark of the sandalwood tree and use it to paint on bindis before prayer.

DESIGNS AND SYMBOLISM

Symbolism in Indian culture is extremely important and mehndi is one of the languages used to express it. The designs drawn in henna throughout India and Pakistan are among the most intricate. Popular are paisley patterns with much repetitive line work and little filling in of larger areas. Mehndi painting is often reminiscent of fabric designs in these particular areas of the world.

All symbols start with the seed (*bija*) from which everything grows. There are simple forms, such as a line (*rekha*) and an angle (*kona*), where two straight lines join to reflect the duality of life. The triangle (*trikona*) either points upwards (*purusa*) as an active male symbol representing fire and the ascent to heaven, or downwards (*prakriti*) as a passive female symbol of water and grace descending from heaven.

A star is symbolic of the presence of divinity and hope. The six-pointed star (*satkona*) brings together the male and female to work in perfect harmony. The hexagon shape within the star (*sadbhuja*) is a powerful form reflected in nature, even in the shape of the cells in our bodies. A five-pointed star (*pancakona*) includes the five elements of fire, water, earth, air and the heavens.

The square (*catuskona*) denotes stability, honesty and shelter, and the diamond (*vajra*) symbolizes enlightenment. The octagon (*astakona*) is made with two overlapping squares and symbolizes protection. The cross (*bavari*) represents a reservoir and is a cosmic symbol denoting communication between heaven and earth. When a square is laid over it (*sarvatobhadra*), it represents a temple with doors on all sides.

The swastika is one of the oldest and most complex symbols, and the word means, 'it is well'. In India, a swastika represents movement, happiness and good fortune, and is often used as a seal on jars of holy water.

The circle is a universal symbol denoting wholeness, but in India its specific meaning is the round of existence in the phenomenal world. A flaming circle is a symbol of *prakriti*, which means, 'that which evolves, produces and brings forth'.

In the Hindu religion, the crescent moon is a newborn baby, quick and eager for growth. The sun is the world door – an entrance to knowledge and immortality. The mandala is a symbol of enlightenment and is usually drawn in the shape of a circle with squares, triangles and circles within the outline. The sun denotes all-seeing divinity and power, with rays that bring life to the world.

The lotus is associated with many symbols, including the bounty in the earth, the tree of life and the female sex organ. The flower usually grows in muddy, marshy water, yet somehow remains pure and clean. It is therefore a symbol of survival in the most challenging surroundings, and Indian philosophy encourages children to be like a lotus, as a dirty environment is not seen as an excuse to become dirty or bad.

Many other flowers and fruits are used as joyful symbols. Flowers portray the fragile quality of childhood and a new life, and fruits, the essence of immortality. Both a rose and an unripe mango (a symbol of virginity) are common for bridal designs. A vine is the symbol of devotion, as it grows towards the light and needs support.

The most common animal design in India is the peacock, which is seen as a companion for a wife during separations from her husband. It is also a symbol of love and desire, since peacocks come out during the rainy season in India – a time of passion. Peacocks are often painted on a bride as a symbol of her forthcoming wedding night. Other birds, such as swans (success) and parrots (the messengers), are popular. Small dots representing falling rain (*bundakis*) symbolize the love a woman shows her husband, while waves (*lahariya*) denote passion and longing.

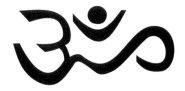

Om (the purest and eternal voice from within, Hindu)

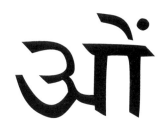

Om (the purest and eternal voice from within, Hindu)

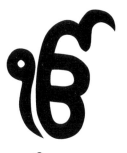

Ek onkar (there is one God, Sikh)

Khanda (Sikh)

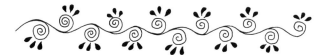

Vine

NORTH AFRICA

*I*n Morocco, henna parties are reminiscent of the culture of hamam – a bathhouse harem where women would lounge around, often naked, and gossip and eat. The parties can last up to three days and are the sole territory of women. Against a backdrop of music, fragrance and food, the atmosphere is lively and sociable. Much excitement and high drama, fuelled with a dose of voodoo-like magic, abounds. The highlight is when the hostess of the party gyrates while in a trance-like state, when the spirit of a jinni is said to enter her body.

Geometric patterns, such as triangles, diamonds and squares, and bold borders (below) are among the most popular designs used by Moroccan women.

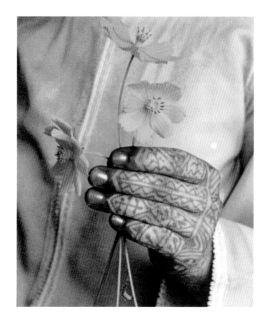

Simple vine patterns painted along each finger (right) accentuate their length and contrast with the elaborate patterns on the hand and the fingertips.

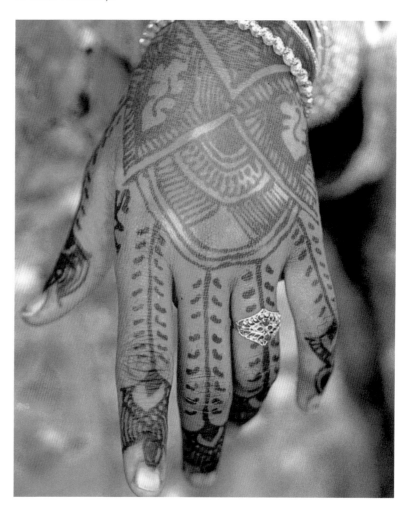

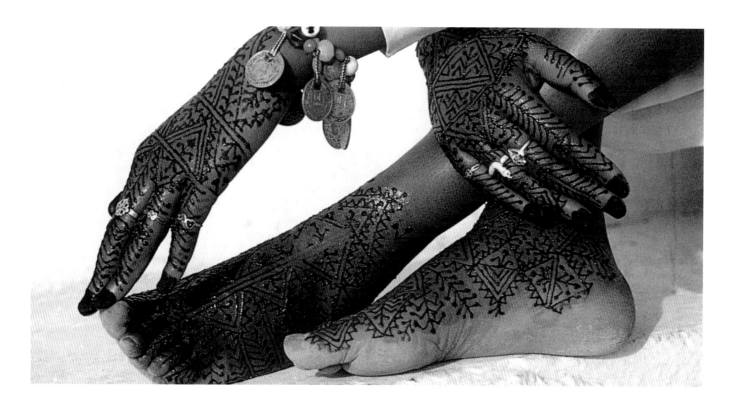

Dancers use mehndi and jewellery to accentuate their hands and feet. In a ritual dance of love called the *Geudra*, the mehndi designs are intended to draw a man's eye towards the flowing movement of the dancer's fingers.

The bold graphic style of North African mehndi patterns enhances the hands and feet, making a bride all the more attractive to her groom.

WEDDING CUSTOMS

Like India, Morocco incorporates mehndi into its wedding ceremonies, but the groom also has a henna gathering on the eve of the wedding. His mother provides an egg, a bottle of water, henna and four candles as a blessing. The groom mixes the egg, water and henna to make a paste, then applies it to his hands. The candles are lit and put in a bowl, and attendants dance around the groom, taking turns to balance the bowl on their heads. They continue until the bowl falls and breaks.

A bride's hair is often soaked with henna paste on her wedding day, and as the women apply it, they sing about the plant of joy, ensuring the bride will run her new house happily. In Morocco, a bride does not automatically live with her husband's family, but seven months after the wedding she must go to visit her in-laws. This is a joyous occasion when she receives many gifts as well as mehndi. A year later, she must visit again, and this time a symbol of stability is drawn in her palm with henna.

A pregnant woman visits a henna artist, known as a *hannayas*, in her seventh month. She receives symbols painted on her ankle and a corresponding amulet, which are thought to protect mother and child throughout the rest of pregnancy and during birth. When the baby is born, a mixture of henna, water and flour is painted over the baby's newly cut belly button to signify a promise of beauty and wealth.

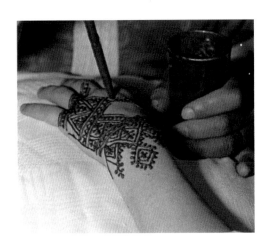

Henna, applied the original way using the tip of a stick, decorates the back of a hand. The modern method is to use a cone applicator (see page 51).

BERBERS AND MEHNDI

The way of life of the Berbers, the indigenous, mainly Muslim people of North Africa, has remained largely unchanged for centuries. They believe in the supernatural and the positive power of the saints, known as *baraka*. The henna plant, among others, is thought to be full of *baraka*, and the main purpose of the mehndi patterns that have been passed through the generations is to protect the wearer from evil spirits.

Berbers believe that anyone going through a transitional stage of life – puberty, marriage, pregnancy or childbirth – is in a weakened state and must be protected from illness and death. Spirits are believed to enter the body through its orifices, especially the eyes, so women use mehndi to protect their faces, hands, feet and any other part of the body not covered by clothing. When a soldier goes to war, his wife applies henna to his right palm to protect him and remind him of her love.

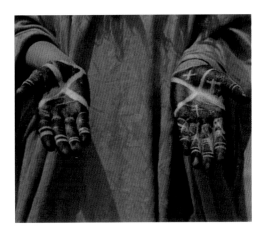

A young girl from Marrakech displays dark and symbolic patterns designed to protect her.

In Morocco, women use permanent tattoos to mark significant occasions in their lives and henna is painted over the top to darken and heal these markings. Many women have the symbol of an eye within a heart painted in the centre of their palm, which is intended to protect their loved ones and make them resist the temptations of other women. Because mehndi is closely connected to love, a widow is not allowed to use henna for four months following the death of her husband, and is also discouraged from taking part in any henna gatherings in the future.

Ironically, henna also plays an important part in death. When a man dies, henna is sprinkled over his head; a woman's hands and feet are painted in mehndi to promote happiness in the next life. Often, mourners dip their hands in henna paste at a funeral to help them come to terms with their loss and the reason for the death.

DESIGNS AND SYMBOLISM

Moroccan women are interested in the magical properties of symbols and their ability to promote fertility and offer protection. The fear-inducing evil eye is blamed for most misfortunes; the motifs used in mehndi are designed to defend against the eye and its negative powers.

There is a repertoire of designs that have been used for centuries, including magic numbers and squares, Arabic script, verses of the Koran, human hands and eyes, and floral motifs. Geometric figures such as triangles, squares, crosses, eight-pointed stars, circles and spirals are also widely used. A popular symbol of the Berbers is a cross at the centre of two diamonds. A diamond (*timrit*) deflects away the evil eye, and one inside the other (*tit*) with a cross at its centre is believed to direct the energy away in four directions.

Basic shapes change their meaning when drawn together. One triangle symbolizes an eye, but five together show a hand. A square is seen to have healing powers; squares joined together symbolize protection. Numerology also influences symbolism, and the number five is particularly important and significant. Wearing this number is thought to give protection, and any combination of five elements is representative of the hand (*khamsa*) of Fatima, daughter of the prophet Mohammed. The serpent is a complex symbol, which in Africa represents a royal emblem, a sign of immortality and incarnations of the dead. The celestial serpent is also a rainbow and either guards the earth's treasures or encircles the earth, quenching its thirst in the sea. Palm branches and date palms symbolize fertility and are traditionally used by a young girl in puberty as a positive sign of the children she hopes to bear in the future.

Most mehndi designs in North Africa are confined to the hands and feet to accentuate their elegant shapes. The most popular design is floral, often geometric in style, and similar to the designs seen in wood carvings, textiles and paintings in the region. Borders with sharp, bold designs are also popular.

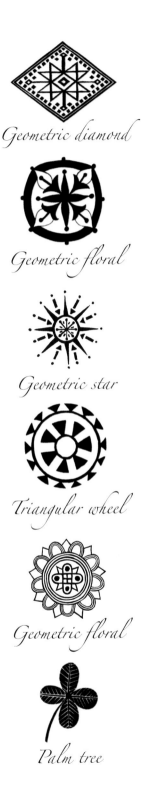

Geometric diamond

Geometric floral

Geometric star

Triangular wheel

Geometric floral

Palm tree

THE MIDDLE EAST

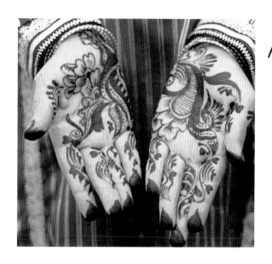

Typically floral in design, the patterns on the palms of a Middle Eastern woman (above) make good use of henna's light and dark tones.

*T*races of henna found on the hands of five-thousand-year-old mummies suggest that mehndi dates back to ancient Egypt. An old Arab proverb says, 'If I don't speak the truth, I don't present my hand for henna', indicating the importance of mehndi in the Middle East, where it is used for decoration and to ward off evil spirits and dangerous spiritual forces.

Henna was also used as a cosmetic in Lower Egypt by privileged women who spent hours beautifying themselves with henna made from the Egyptian evergreen plant *Lawsonia inermis*. Staining the nails, skin and hair with henna remains a popular beauty trick of the Middle East. Mehndi is not the only beauty trend to come out of Egypt; many modern cosmetic treatments originated there, including perms, hair extensions and wigs, and the basics of Western make-up – eye shadow, kohl pencil and lipstick – were originally used by the pampered women of ancient Egypt.

The use of mehndi in wedding ceremonies in the Middle East is crucial, and the traditions surrounding the art are similar to those followed in India. Women gather a few days before the wedding to decorate the bride's hands and feet with henna designs. The hours are filled with excitement, singing and much teasing of the bride.

Fluid and fanciful, these flower motifs (right) match but are not identical; much of the flesh is deliberately left exposed to heighten the effect.

A bride from Oman (opposite) embellishes her patterned hands with heavy bracelets and red-painted nails, thickly outlined with henna.

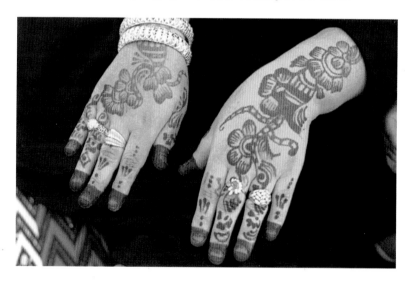

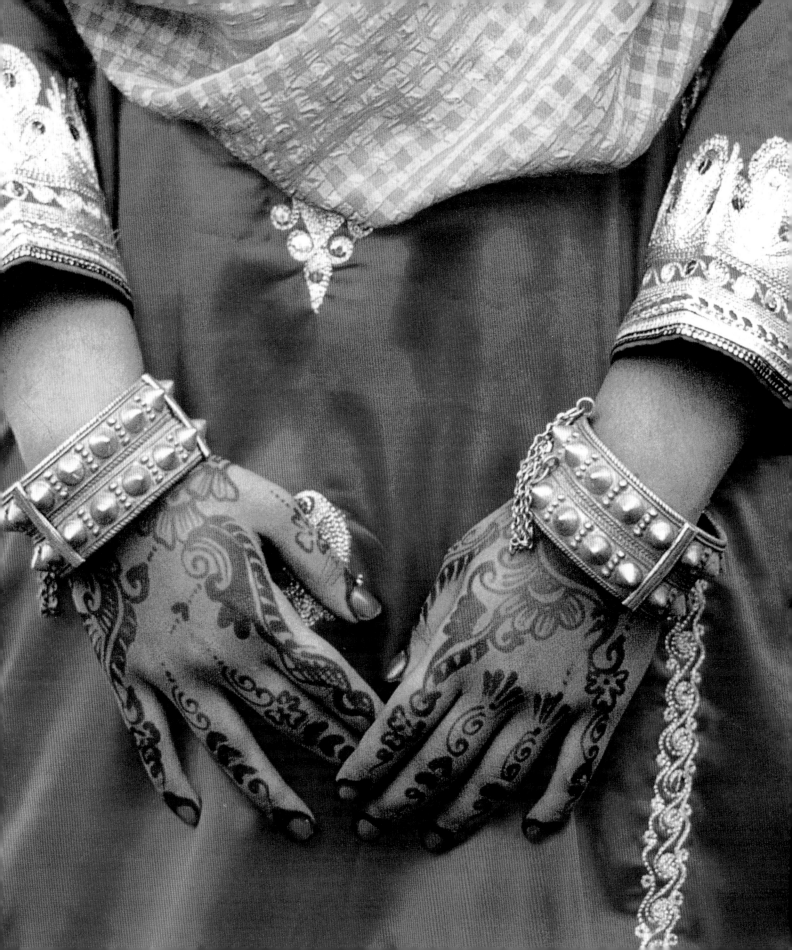

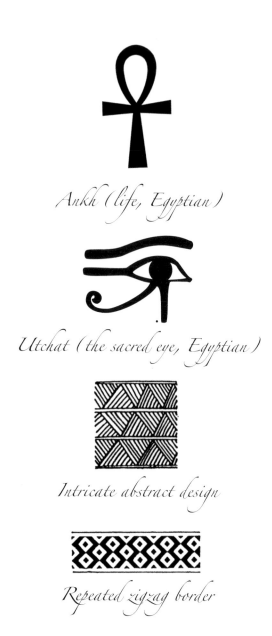

Ankh (life, Egyptian)

Utchat (the sacred eye, Egyptian)

Intricate abstract design

Repeated zigzag border

Enclosed vertical spirals

DESIGNS AND SYMBOLISM

Influenced by the patterns used in Arabic carvings, textiles and paintings, the designs of Middle Eastern mehndi are mostly floral. Typically, they are built up around a centrepiece with plenty of space left unadorned to allow the flesh to show through. On special occasions, such as weddings and feasts, women embellish themselves further by dying their nails a deep red to match and enhance their intricate mehndi designs. For day wear, Bedouin women apply henna in simple, basic shapes with no definite pattern. They colour the entire sole of the foot or palm of the hand, filling in the finger and toe tips completely.

In Egypt, the right eye symbolizes the sun and the left eye symbolizes the moon. The moon is usually represented as the feminine power with the sun as the masculine opposite. A moon is universally symbolic of the rhythm of time, and in Egypt it represents the maker of eternity and the creator of all things everlasting. The sun is the supreme cosmic force with all-seeing divinity and power.

The lizard is believed to be tongueless and to exist on dew, and as such, in mehndi designs it is a symbol of silence. Egyptians also believe the lizard represents divine wisdom and good fortune. A winged circle symbolizes the rising sun, and a veil is 'the universe which the goddess weaves'.

Much Egyptian decoration, however, is not symbolic. One of the first popular shapes was the zigzag line, either symmetrically doubled or repeated in borders in alternate light and dark colours. This pattern was originally inspired by textile designs, and later, it became a rounded wavy line. In Egyptian mehndi, the popular lotus motif is considered a thing of beauty, rather than a sacred plant. Second only to the lotus in importance is the spiral, which is said to symbolize the wanderings of the soul. These three designs were the first ornaments of importance in Egypt, and feathers and flowers followed later.

SOUTH-EAST ASIA

Although it is not practised so widely in Islamic South-East Asia, mehndi is still an important part of a wedding ceremony. The female's age at marriage is highly significant as it reflects her entry into the household, as well as her childbearing and sexual responsibilities. A combination of superstition and religion ensures that anything considered to be a good omen, such as mehndi, is taken seriously. As in India, it is believed that the longer the wedding mehndi stains last, the more the mother-in-law will love her son's bride, encouraging her to make her henna last as long as possible.

DESIGNS AND SYMBOLISM

Mehndi designs are similar to those in India, although they are usually less detailed and cover a smaller area of skin. They also have much in common with Middle Eastern designs in that the finger and toe tips are completely coloured in with henna, and there is often a solid circle around the whole of the lower foot.

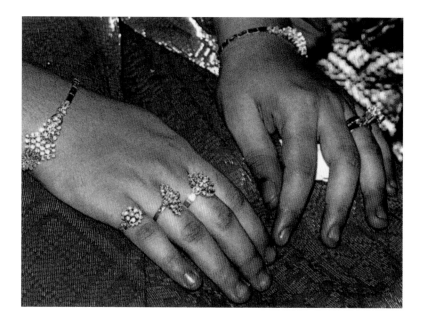

Often South-East Asian brides dye only the tips of their fingers with henna and go to great lengths to preserve the colour of the stains.

HENNA

For centuries the natural conditioning and dyeing properties of the henna plant have been used to treat and colour the hair. The bright-green shrub-like plant (*Lawsonia inermis*) originates from Egypt where it thrives in the country's hot, dry climate. Henna is also grown in India, the Sudan, North Africa and the Middle East. However, the plant is best suited to tropical climates and grows well in a greenhouse. Henna has the potential to grow to 4.6 metres (15 feet), but never reaches its full height as it is harvested at between 2.4 metres (8 feet) and 3 metres (10 feet), three times a year.

Henna is the Persian name for this flowering shrub with small leaves and thick bark. Other names include henne, Al-Khanna, Al-henna, Jamaica Mignonette, Egyptian Privet and Smooth Lawsonia. The flower is delicate, with four petals and elongated stamen protruding from the centre. The red, rose-pink and white blossoms have a sweet honey-like scent, similar to jasmine, rose and mignonette, and the flower's oil has been used for centuries as a perfume.

HARVESTING HENNA

Harvesting begins as soon as the flowers appear. The plant is cut as close to its base as possible and the branches are broken off and left in the sun for two days to dry. The leaves from the top shoots contain the strongest dye, so these are separated and dried first to ensure little loss of colour. These make the highest grade henna powder, used exclusively for staining the skin. The rest of the leaves are dried and shaken off the branches. These are destined for cheaper hair dyes, shampoos and conditioners.

Many customers prefer to buy henna in its original leaf form to be sure it has not been mixed with any other plants. It is also cheaper to buy the leaves and grind them at home, usually with a pestle and mortar. Pre-ground henna is often bought by more affluent buyers for export purposes. Sacks of leaves are taken to a local generally caused

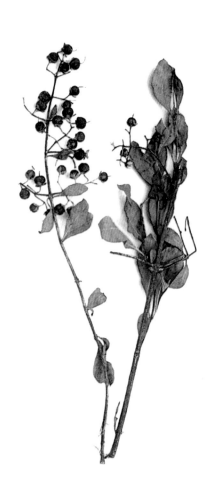

The small, round green leaves and berry-like seeds of the henna plant (Lawsonia inermis). The plant has numerous names and varieties.

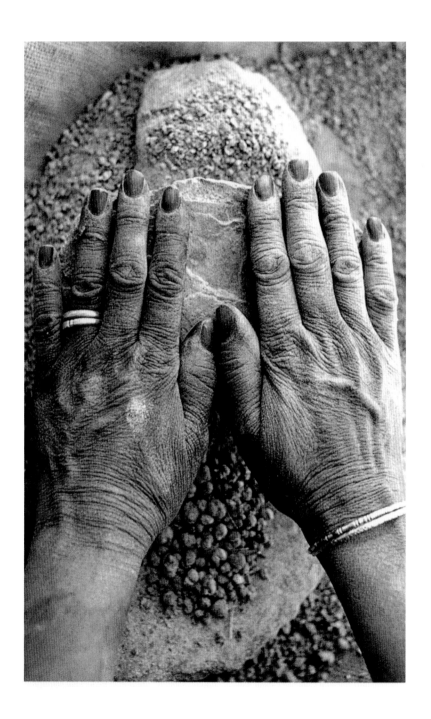

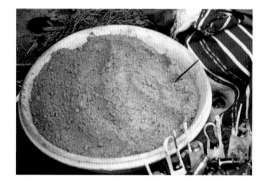

Vivid green and freshly crushed, raw henna powder (above) goes on sale at a Moroccan market stall.

A woman grinds henna into a powder between two rocks (above left). The fine dusting of henna powder that covers her hands keeps them cool as she works.

by transportation. The final stage is to sieve the powder before sending it to manufacturing companies for packaging. The more the henna powder is sieved, the stronger the stain it creates.

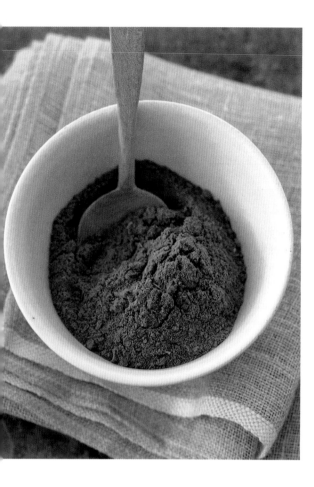

The finer the henna powder, the deeper the colour.

EARLY HISTORY OF HENNA

Henna is probably the most widely used cosmetic of all time. Archaeologists have discovered henna on the hair and nails of Egyptian mummies, suggesting that the earliest evidence of henna dates back to around 1200 BC. Apparently, it was common for Egyptians to colour their fingernails with henna, and not to sport reddish stained nails was thought to be bad mannered.

The great prophet Mohammed was said to dye his hair and beard with henna, which popularized the practice in Saudi Arabia around the year 632 BC. Not to be left out, Muslim women also stained their hands and feet.

Henna travelled from Egypt to India, and the first Indian queen said to have been painted with the paste was the wife of Emperor Shah Jahan, Mumtaz Mahal, for whom the Taj Mahal was built.

HENNA AS A HEALER

The desert people of Rajasthan, Punjab and Gujarat were the first to stumble upon the cooling properties of the henna plant. They found that by dipping their hands and feet in a paste made from the crushed leaves gave them much needed relief from the unremitting heat. They also noticed that once the paste had been scraped off, as long as the colour remained, so did the cooling effect. Women began painting one large central dot in the palm of their hands, sometimes with smaller dots added around it, and found that this had the same result. This encouraged them to start creating designs, applying the paste with a thin piece of silver, ivory or wood. These instruments were the same as those used to apply kohl around the eyes, and the type that are still used in some desert villages today.

Long known for its many healing properties, henna is a particularly popular treatment for skin disorders in India and North Africa. An efficient antiseptic and astringent, it is often used to make an instant 'scab' over open wounds and can also soothe burns and eczema. Henna also provides relief from bruises and sprains as well as rheumatic and arthritic pain. Because of its cooling effect, henna can be mixed with vinegar and applied to the head to help relieve a headache. Henna on the feet can also soothe a headache (often caused by heat), and it is also used as a cure for athlete's foot, corns, foot odour, blisters and minor cuts. The palm of the hand contains so many nerve endings that if a ball of henna paste is held, it helps reduce a fever. Long used as a conditioner, to prevent hair loss, kill head lice and cure dandruff, henna has also been known to work wonders on illnesses such as leprosy, smallpox, jaundice and even certain cancers.

Sackfuls of dried henna leaves attract buyers who are prepared to grind the leaves themselves, either by hand or at a local mill.

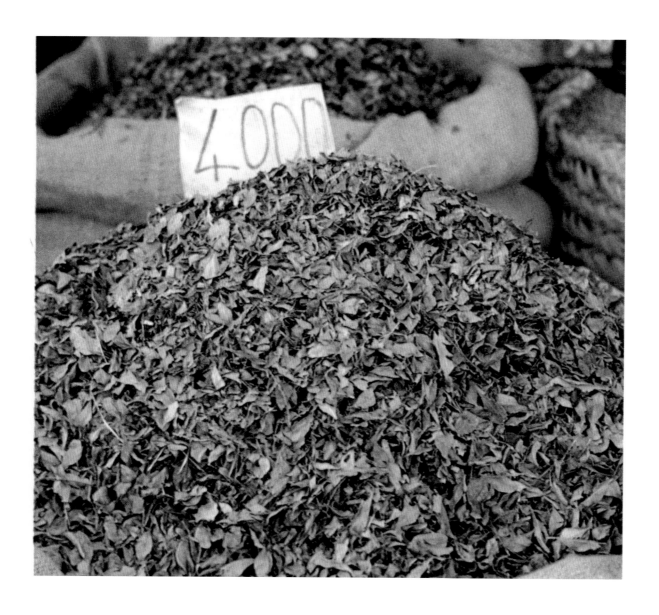

With all things Eastern making their mark throughout the Western world – from holistic therapies to styles of dress – it follows naturally that mehndi has become a must-have fashion accessory.

Many stars are fans of the look, and as with most trends that are adopted by celebrities, the art of mehndi has attracted an enthusiastic following. Actress Liv Tyler's arms were painted in 'lace gloves' and photographed by celebrity snapper Herb Ritts for the cover of *Vanity Fair* magazine. Madonna had her hands and feet decorated for the video of her 1998 comeback single 'Frozen'. Demi Moore, Gwen Stefani and Naomi Campbell have all been seen wearing henna tattoos together with bindis and original Indian saris to fashionable events in Los Angeles, New York and Paris.

How ironic, then, that this Western interpretation of an Eastern practice is championed by the rich and famous, when traditionally mehndi was developed and worn by poor women who, unable to afford elaborate jewellery, turned to this cheap and natural alternative way of adorning their bodies for special occasions.

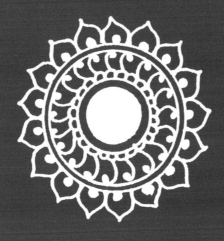

Chapter 2

THE WESTERN WORLD

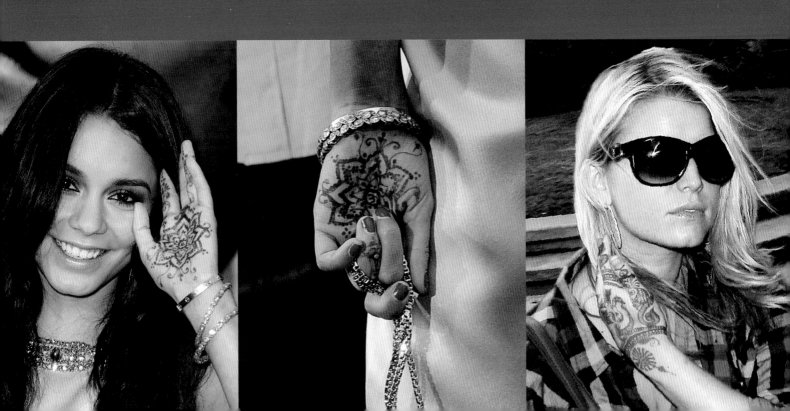

MEHNDI GROWS TRENDY

The new trend for everything Eastern shows a shift in Western thinking away from the material towards the spiritual. With the West already interested in many ancient metaphysical therapies, the appeal of mehndi is not just in decorating the body, but as a holistic experience to share.

Public interest in mehndi began to grow in 1996 when Lorretta Roome, a musician, met Indian artist Rani Patel in New York. Under Rani's teachings, Lorretta learnt the art of mehndi and held a photographic exhibition to demonstrate it in a gallery in the city. The exhibition attracted immense media attention, particularly because of the temporary nature of the henna art form.

At the same time, stylist L'Wren Scott discovered my beauty centre, Ziba, the oldest and largest Indian beauty salon on the West coast. The salon is well known because it is situated close to Los Angeles in the heart of Little India in the city of Artesia – home to the second largest group of Indian businesses in the United States.

L'Wren Scott had her hands and feet painted with traditional mehndi. When she attended a number of high-profile parties in Hollywood adorned with the tattoos she received much attention and appreciation for the henna paintings. She then went on to hire Ziba to paint the hands and feet of actress Liv Tyler, who was photographed by Herb Ritts for the cover of *Vanity Fair*. The issue hit the newsstands in April 1997, and soon afterwards features on the art of mehndi followed in many of the major fashion and beauty magazines, and on television.

All the attention mehndi received was due to two main factors. Where Hollywood goes, the rest of us soon follow, and there was no shortage of stars who wanted to be seen wearing mehndi. Demi Moore, Mira Sorvino, the artist formerly known as Prince and Naomi Campbell all appeared at high-profile events wearing the tattoos. The second important factor in mehndi's growth was its temporary and painless status. Tattoos that last up to three weeks were the perfect alternative to the other hot trend of the moment – painful and permanent tattoos.

Vanessa Hudgens and Jessica Simpson (previous page) are some of the young Hollywood celebrities sporting mehndi designs.

Actress Liv Tyler (far right) was photographed by Herb Ritts for Vanity Fair in 1997.

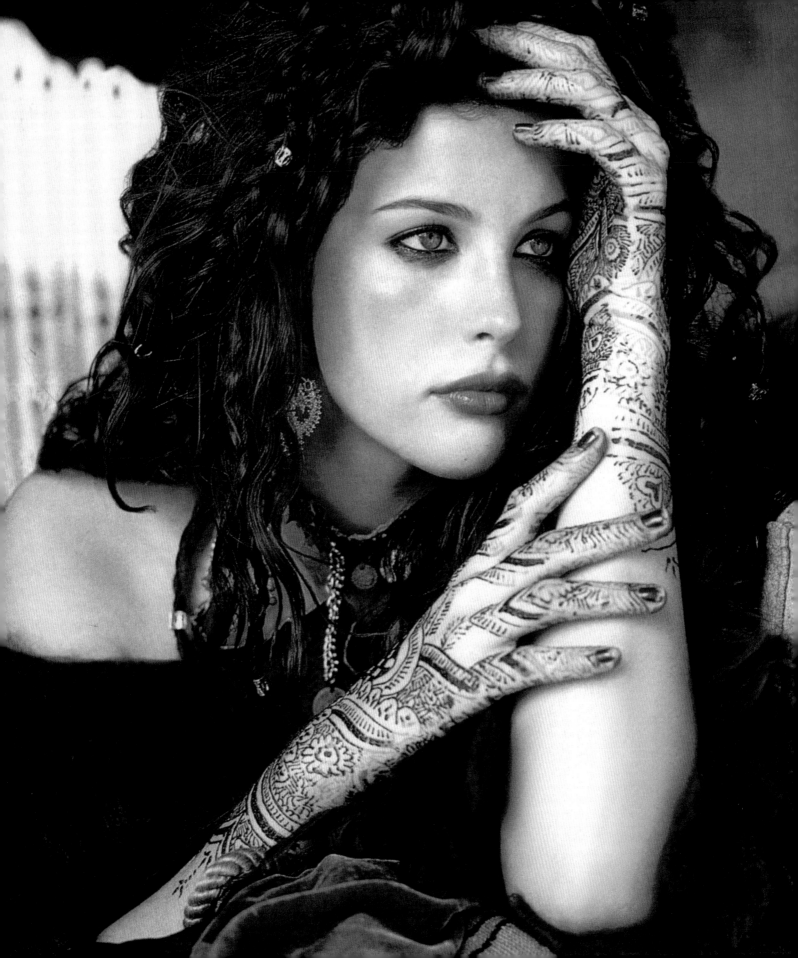

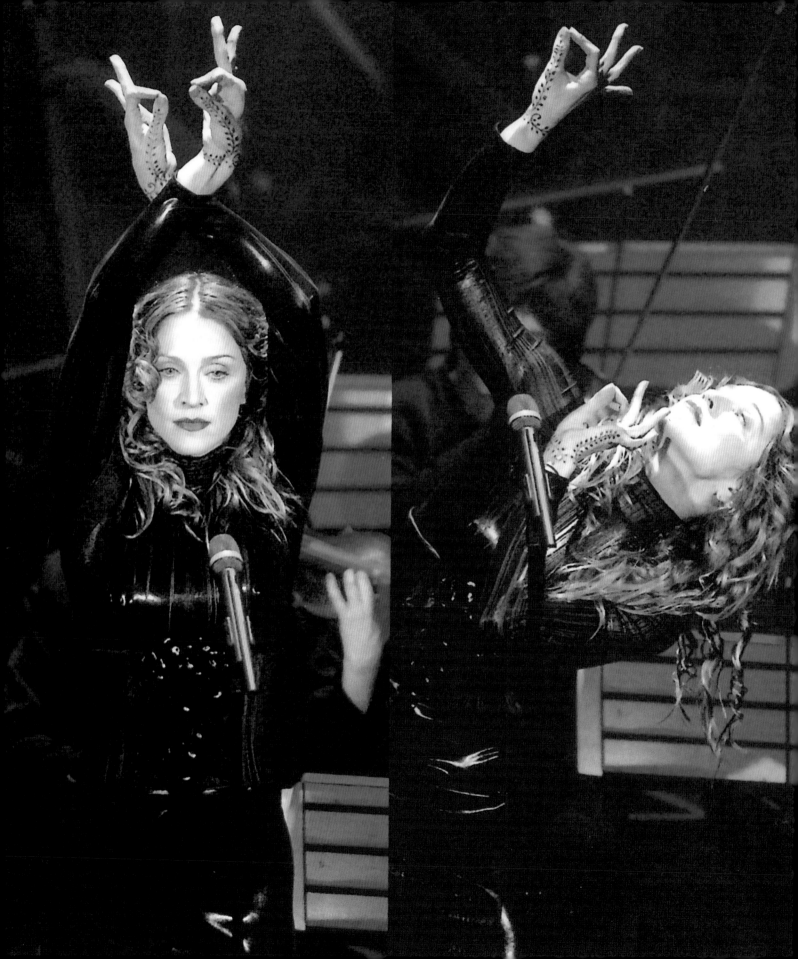

One star who helped put mehndi on the map was Gwen Stefani, lead singer of American band No Doubt. Her meteoric rise to fame, following the release of the ballad 'Don't Speak', made her a star whose style was suddenly under scrutiny. With her passion for mehndi, bindis and beautiful bright saris, she was guaranteed to be photographed wherever she put in an appearance.

However, it is Madonna who is perhaps mehndi's most high-profile admirer. Consistent with her uncanny talent for pioneering new trends, she embraced the art to complement her new spiritual awareness of the 1990s. Having abandoned her boned corsets and bleached blonde crop for flowing fabrics and a mass of tangled curls, henna-painted hands and feet completed the star's caring, serene attitude in accordance with her new single-mother lifestyle in the late 1990s.

It all began in December 1997, when I was contacted by world-famous make-up artist Joanne Gair, who had been responsible for body painting Demi Moore in a tuxedo for a cover of *Vanity Fair*, along with numerous other credits to her name. Madonna had asked Joanne to find a mehndi artist to decorate her hands and feet for a video for her new single 'Frozen'. When it was released in the January of the following year, the whole world was suddenly introduced to the temporary tattoo art form. To guarantee even more coverage, Madonna appeared all over the United States and Europe wearing henna paintings for the promotion of her single, and the media eulogized her ability to set trends in motion.

Soon after, I was contacted by model Naomi Campbell, actress Peggy Lipton, singer Aliyah and many other celebrities to paint them with henna. I have also had the privilege of painting actress Jennifer Aniston for the cover of *US* magazine, and I appeared on British television on Channel 4's 'The Big Breakfast', where I painted presenters Denise Van Outen and Johnny Vaughan.

Today, henna is in worldwide demand and millions of women have discovered the mystery and mystique of this beautiful herb. Ironically, the adornment of the poorest women of the East, who were unable to afford jewellery, has become the fashion accessory of some of the richest women in the world.

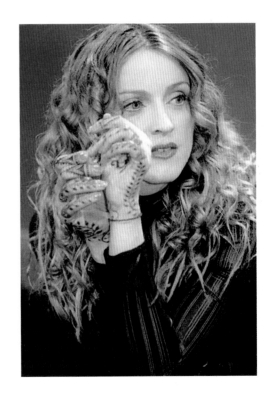

Madonna wears mehndi on her hands for her 1998 single 'Frozen' from the Ray of Light *album (above and opposite).*

FAMOUS DEVOTEES

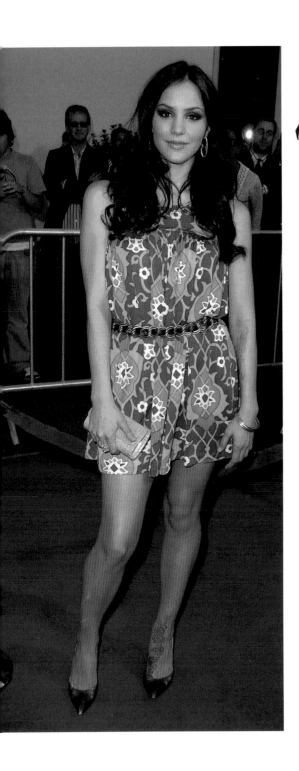

Mira Sorvino had her hands painted for her appearance at the 1997 Oscar awards ceremony. Superstars Demi Moore and the artist formerly known as Prince have also been seen sporting mehndi designs. Among others in the public eye, actresses Neve Campbell, Daryl Hannah and Angela Bassett have been fans, and Gavin Rossdale, lead singer with rock band Bush, has also worn henna tattoos. Sting and his wife Trudi Styler claim that painting henna designs on each other's bodies heightens the therapeutic benefits of mehndi.

Naomi Campbell is among many other top models in the pubic eye who have worn mehndi designs on their hands – despite the fact that the dye lasts for around three weeks. However, it is Madonna, my most high-profile customer, who is truly responsible for bringing the ancient art form under the media spotlight. In addition to wearing mehndi designs on her hands and feet for her 'Frozen' video, she also had intricately painted hands throughout her publicity tours in both America and Britain. Pictures of her at the MTV Music Awards sporting mehndi were guaranteed to give the trend even more celebrity clout. Another pioneer of the trend was Gwen Stefani, lead singer of American band No Doubt, who is a huge fan of all things Eastern and another loyal client of mine. The singer embraced the total look of the East, with everything from body piercing and mehndi to wearing saris and bindis. On many occasions she attended public events and music award ceremonies sporting the complete look.

Singer and actress Katherine McPhee (left)
walked the red carpet after getting painted
at Ziba Beauty in Artesia, California.

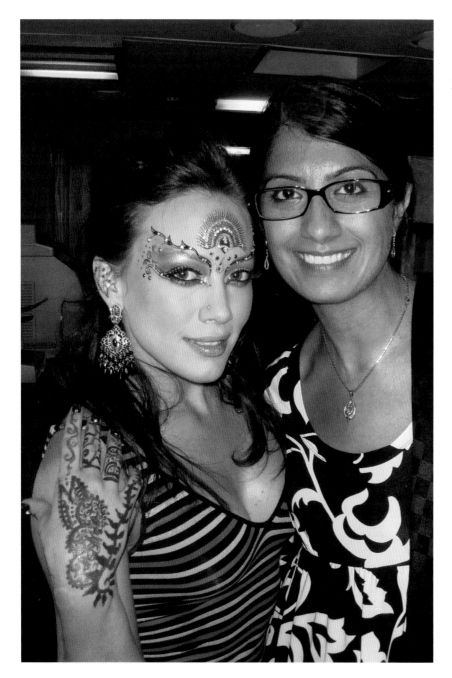

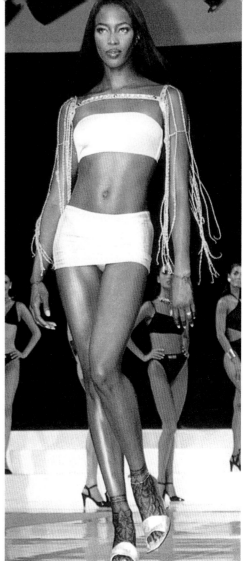

Mehndi enters the world of fashion (above) as Naomi Campbell's decorative feet stride down the catwalk.

Actress Hillary Duff with author Sumita Batra on the set of her music video 'Stranger'.

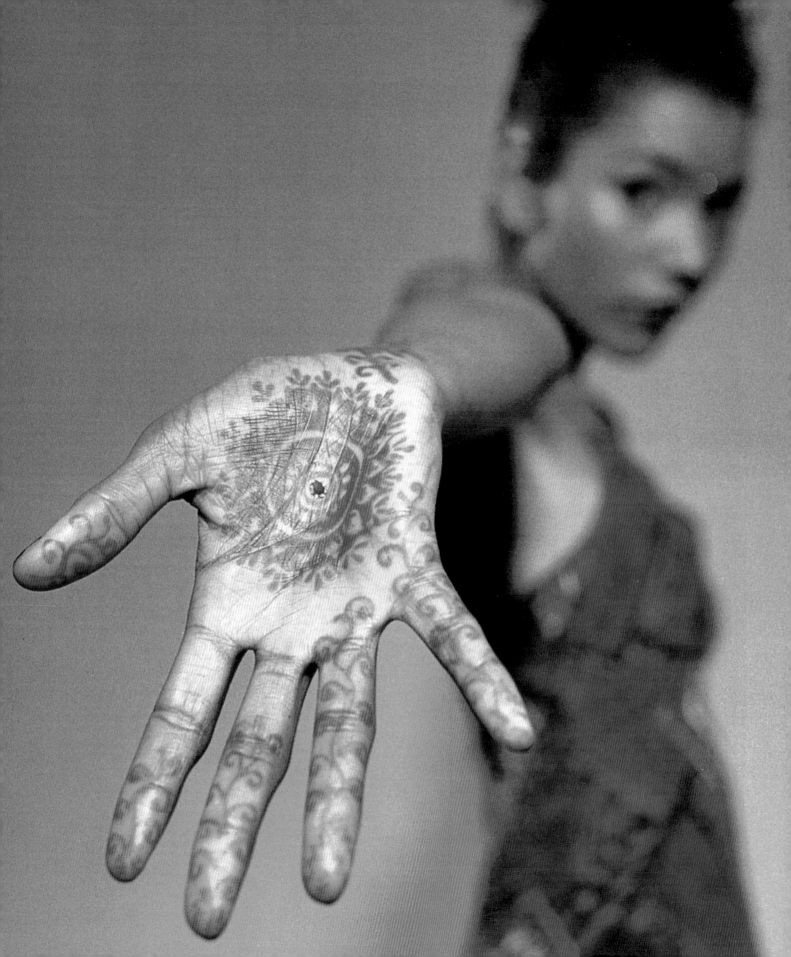

FASHION PACK

Permanent tattoos are often the mark of celebrities who want to show off their individuality. Rihanna, Scarlet Johansson, David Beckham, Megan Fox and countless top models chose to make a statement and colour their bodies for life. However, with those in the public eye always under pressure to reinvent themselves, many find that non-permanent body paints provide the perfect way to change their image in an instant to match a mood or outfit, without drastic consequences.

Whatever styles or trends are seen on the catwalk are guaranteed to be worn by the fashion elite, before they eventually filter down to the high street. Increasingly, fashion shows have revealed models adorned with body paint. In the 1990s, Clements Ribeiro drew Celtic designs on their models, using swirling designs on their backs and arms; Alexander McQueen and Jean Paul Gaultier also accessorized their models with more than just the standard eyeliner and lipstick. In 2010 Rodarte showed girls wearing Maori-inspired geometric body paintings on the catwalk and Chanel launched delicate trompe-l'oeil tattoo transfers on the legs, wrists and necklines of models.

It usually takes more than a single season for a directional catwalk look to filter down to the high street, but body art has proved to be the exception. Major chain stores and many local high street retailers stock their shelves with non-permanent tattoo-painting and mehndi kits that are easy to use and suitable for all ages.

Mehndi is not a mere fad. On the contrary, it provides a long-lasting and spiritual method for adorning the body. It is also an extremely versatile and timeless means of creating a new eye-catching look. Its far-reaching history and the traditions that surround its application will undoubtedly ensure that mehndi is a favourite form of body decoration for the fashion pack.

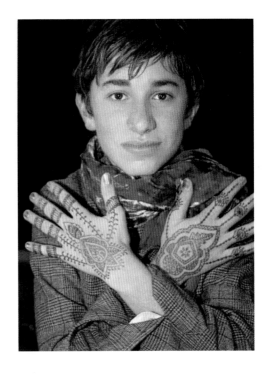

American fashion designer Todd Oldham (above) proves that creative hands deserve special treatment and that mehndi is not restricted to women alone.

Up close and personal, mehndi commands the attention of the camera (left) and has made a permanent mark in the fashion world.

White body paint can be used on the forehead to emphasize the impact of a single bindi, or worked in delicate dots and swirls to imitate the effect of lace on bare skin. Both approaches add a new Eastern dimension to the traditional dress of a Western bride. Modern mehndi designs such as these can be painted in any shade to coordinate with the bride's and her attendants' clothing and accessories.

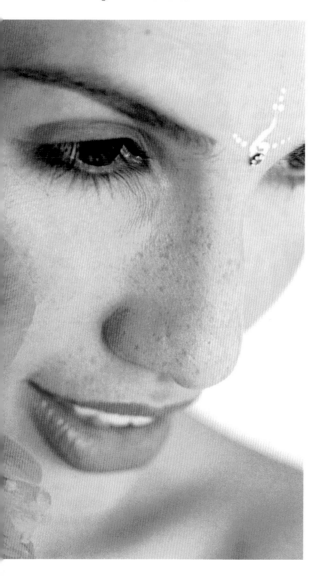

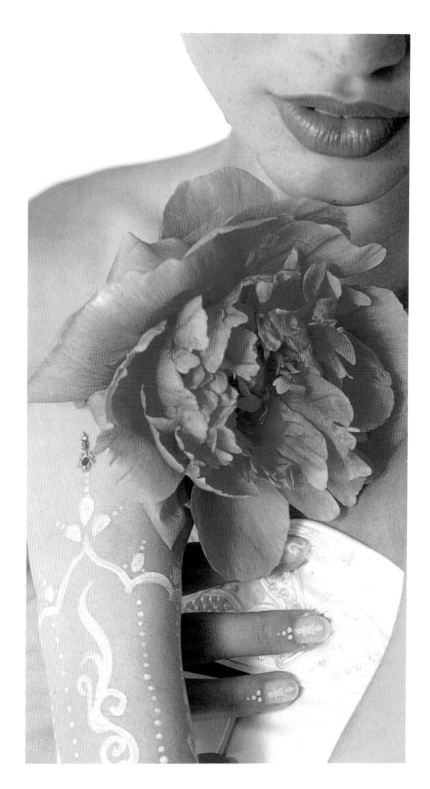

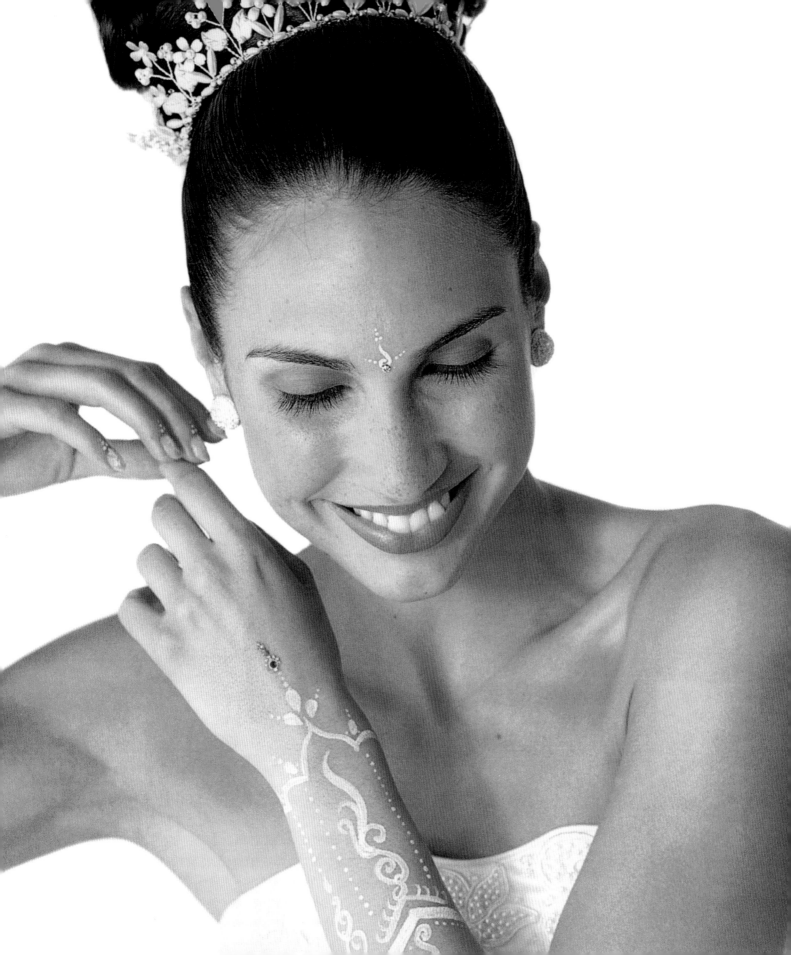

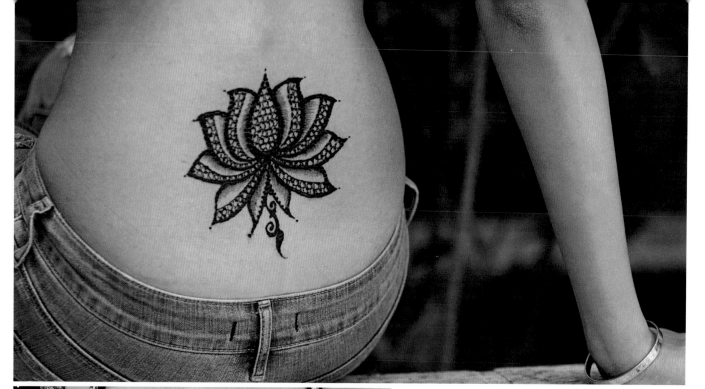

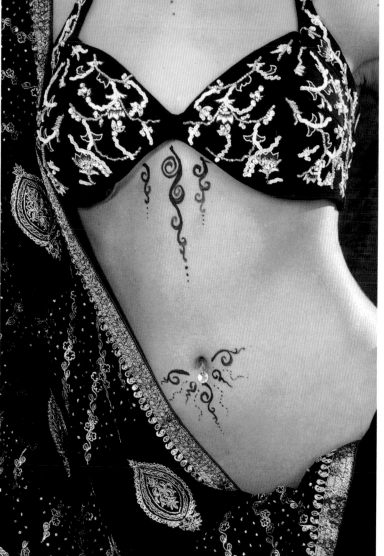

Today, Mehndi has taken its own Western interpretation and is being adorned on the body as an accessory in the same places as permanent tattoos are usually positioned – the centre lower back (above), the tummy button (left) and the upper arm (right).

WHERE TO WEAR

*T*he fashionable trendsetters among us may have enthusiastically embraced Indian traditions, but Western women choose to paint their mehndi decorations on areas of the body that Asian women would never contemplate. In the West, the belly button seems to be the most popular place for a henna ring, while the back offers an expansive canvas for larger and more intricate designs. These are both areas of the body that are definitely out of bounds for traditional mehndi wearers.

Henna decorations and symbols are an alternative to permanent tattoos, which have been so popular with models and pop stars in recent years. Favourite places for tattoos, such as the ankles, wrists, hip bone and the base of the spine, were always the most sensitive areas under the tattooist's needle, but these areas can be quickly and painlessly painted with henna. With a life expectancy of only three weeks, mehndi tattoos offer a risk-free opportunity to experiment with a tattoo before taking the plunge and going for the indelible option.

Initially, women are attracted to mehndi primarily because of the temporary nature of the henna tattoos, but when they learn a little more about the history of mehndi, the cultural significance of the henna herb and its power to heal, the ancient art form takes on a far more important meaning. Its significance is now recognized to such an extent in the West that it is becoming an important part of many bridal and baby showers.

In the back-to-basics culture in which we live, another significant attraction for many mehndi devotees is that henna is a completely natural product, which – unless you have an allergy to it – has no health risks. On the contrary, it has many benefits apart from the merely decorative, being a natural antiseptic and astringent, which cleanses the skin of impurities. It also works as a total sun block and can help to relieve certain skin conditions and act as a conditioner that will leave the skin feeling supple, soft and smooth.

The traditional art form in a modern fashion context (below) reveals mehndi's timeless quality and lasting beauty.

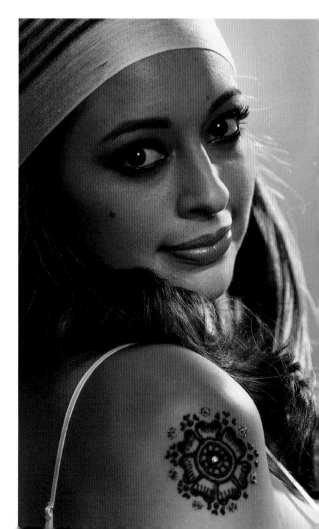

Anyone who can doodle on a piece of paper can create their own mehndi designs. All you need is the patience and time to perfect your drawings, make the henna paste and improve your technique.

Before you do anything else, it is important to practise your design and make sure you are completely happy with it, since once the henna has been applied you will have to live with the tattoo for up to three weeks. Before you make the paste, it is also a good idea to try painting with toothpaste, which has a similar texture and consistency to henna paste. Keep practising until you have a steady and confident hand.

The process of mehndi is not just about creating beautiful designs on your body. Traditionally mehndi was a prelude to an important celebration, so treat the process as a relaxing and therapeutic experience. After all, when else do you have the excuse to sit still for so long? Take a tip from Eastern brides, and even if you can't avoid doing the housework until the henna decoration fades, at least allow yourself an indulgent rest while you wait for the paste to penetrate.

Chapter 3

HOW TO APPLY HENNA

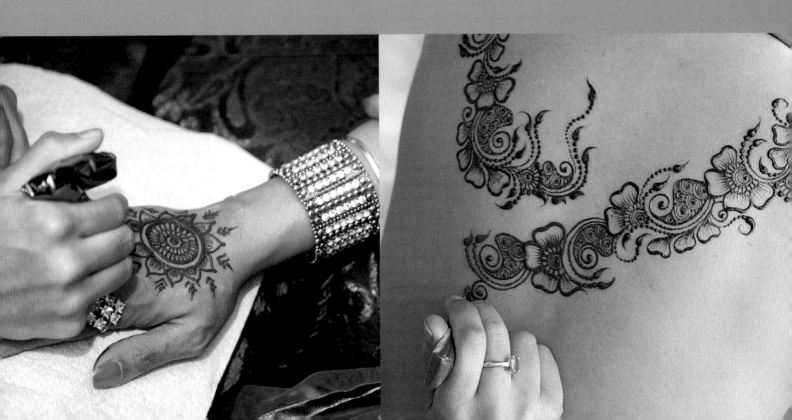

HENNA

There is a big difference between the quality of henna that is for use on the hair and the type manufactured for staining the skin. For body painting, don't buy the type made for use on hair because it is not strong enough to stain your skin and it may also contain added ingredients, such as metal salts to encourage the henna to penetrate the hair shaft. Hair henna is usually coarser than skin-quality henna and is often grey-brown or dark green in colour. Henna of any other colour may have had dyes added and will not have the same staining power and may cause allergic reactions. Most important is to steer clear of black henna, which often contains chemicals and can cause serious skin reactions. What you should look for is bright green, finely ground henna powder. As a rule, the brighter the colour, the deeper its stain will be. Top-quality henna smells fragrant like a fresh herb, so use your nose to sniff out a good mehndi product and avoid anything with an unpleasant, toxic smell. You should be able to find quality henna in health-food shops, pharmacies, drugstores, specialist beauty shops and Indian and Moroccan stores. Beware of promises of 'pure henna' – it is worth checking the colour and smell before buying. Pre-made pastes are also slightly suspect, as real henna paste will only stay fresh for up to four days. This means ready-made products must contain preservatives, which can diminish the beneficial effects to the skin. Always make your own henna paste if you have the time.

Remember that what starts out as good-quality henna may deteriorate due to poor packaging. For this reason, you must always keep your henna in an airtight container away from direct sunlight. If it is exposed to light, it will begin to bleach, which diminishes its staining power. Similarly, if it is exposed to air, the water vapour in the atmosphere will start to activate the powder and it will begin to dye itself.

Pure henna is a safe, natural product, which rarely causes an allergic reaction. Although ingesting it will not harm you, it is not advisable to take it internally, since the powder may affect your red blood cells and cause temporary jaundice.

PREPARING YOUR SKIN

Your henna designs will last longer if you exfoliate your skin the day before application, either with a scrub product or a loofah. Once the dead surface layer of cells has been removed, the henna stain can 'fix' on to a new smooth layer of skin. If the area you are decorating is hairy, remove the hair with a shaver, wax or depilatory cream the day before. (You should avoid doing this on the same day as you may risk irritation.) Don't forget, if you are painting your hands, you will be unable to use them for two to six hours. Make sure you complete any important chores ahead of time so that you can do absolutely nothing with a clear conscience.

Immediately before applying the henna paste, cleanse the area you are about to cover with facial cleansing cream and cotton wool. Then apply alcohol-free toner to remove any leftover grease, which will prevent the henna from being absorbed.

WHAT YOU NEED

To make traditional henna paste, you will need the following ingredients to add to the henna powder:

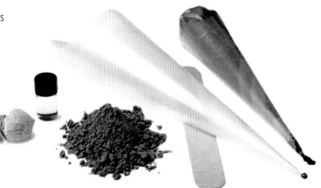

black tea: preferably Indian.

dark coffee: preferably instant.

tamarind paste: an important part of the mixture as it deepens the colour of the stain. It is usually sold dried or as a concentrate.

eucalyptus oil: look for essential oil in a dark glass bottle.

ground cloves: to enhance the colour.

whole cloves: another colour enhancer; the longer you soak them in water, the stronger their effect will be.

lemon and sugar fixer: to set your design (see page 53 for the recipe). The citric acid in the lemon helps the henna soak into the skin and deepen the colour, while the sugar helps the design stick and prevents the henna paste from flaking off before the stain has penetrated the skin.

You will need the following equipment to make up the henna paste:

fine-mesh sieve: even finely ground henna powder should be sieved before use, especially if your design calls for delicate lines. The aim is to have your henna powder as close to the consistency of flour as possible. In India, a white muslin cloth is used, while Moroccan women sometimes use a nylon stocking, stretched over the opening of a bowl or jar. You can use this method at home by securing the stocking in place with a rubber band and pushing the powder through with a spoon. Be prepared for this process to take some time!

mehndi cone: the most common applicator used today in India and the Middle East. The cone resembles a small piping bag and is simple to make (see opposite). All you need is a piece of heavy-duty plastic (a freezer bag is ideal, or a piece of plastic sheeting), some scissors and strong adhesive tape.

cotton-wool buds: to wipe away mistakes and absorb any blobs of paste that ooze out of your mehndi cone.

flat-edged toothpick or manicure stick: to steady uneven lines, or thin down thick ones.

paper tissues: to wipe up as you work.

PATCH TEST

Before making up the henna paste, check that you are not allergic to any of the ingredients required. Using a cotton-wool bud (swab), dab a small amount of each of the substances in turn – including the henna powder itself – on to a patch of skin on the inside of your forearm where the skin is most sensitive. Cover the area with a dressing and wait for 24 hours to check that none of the ingredients has caused any irritation.

Next, test the staining ability of the henna by mixing together a little of the powder and some water. Allow it to stand for an hour and then apply a small dot to the sole of your foot. Wait 10–15 minutes for the henna to dry, then scrape it off. If you are left with a mark, then your henna powder is good quality and it is worth investing all the time and effort required to make and apply the paste.

MAKING A CONE

Creating your own mehndi cone takes practice, so be prepared to attempt it a few times before getting it right. When using the cone, gently squeeze out the henna from the top to avoid bursting the seams.

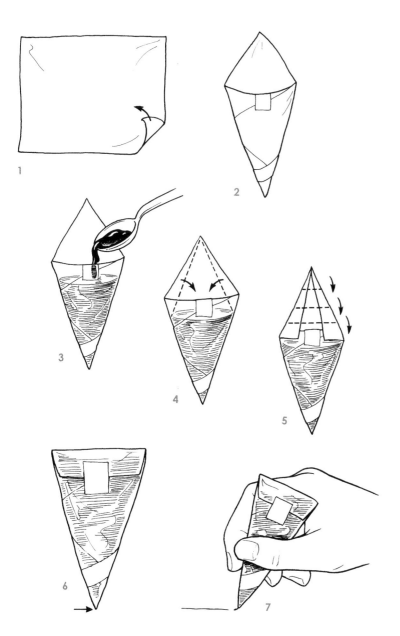

1 Cut a rectangle, 18 x 12.5 cm (7 x 5 in), out of the heavy-duty plastic.

2 Roll the plastic diagonally from one corner inwards to form a funnel or cone with an opening in the tip no thicker than a pin and an opening at the top wide enough to hold two fingers. Use strong adhesive tape to hold the cone in shape and seal the edges.

3 Use a teaspoon to half-fill the cone with henna paste.

4 Fold both sides of the wide end inwards, then downwards.

5 Repeat this several times until the paste is pressed into a compact block.

6 Make sure there is no leakage and seal every seam with another layer of tape so the henna cannot squirt out over your hands.

7 Test your cone to see if the opening in the tip is wide enough to let the henna squeeze out. If it is not, prick the end with a pin or carefully snip it with scissors.

THE BASIC RECIPE

HENNA PASTE

INGREDIENTS

The amount of liquid absorbed by the
henna powder depends on the type of
powder used. The recipe given below is
approximate, and the important thing
is to achieve a paste with the consistency
of toothpaste.

2 tea bags

2 teaspoons coffee

2 teaspoons tamarind paste

1 teaspoon ground cloves

6–8 whole cloves

425 ml (¾ pint) water

5–6 tablespoons henna powder

5 drops eucalyptus oil

EQUIPMENT

old saucepan

fine sieve

mixing bowl

spoon

INSTRUCTIONS

1 Place the tea bags, coffee, tamarind paste and the ground and
whole cloves in the saucepan. Pour in 425 ml (¾ pint) water, mix the
ingredients together and bring it to the boil. Allow the mixture to simmer
for about an hour and then leave it to cool. (The more you boil the
water, the stronger the mix will become.)

2 Sieve the henna powder into a glass, ceramic or stainless steel mixing
bowl. Strain the cooled mixture, add a little and stir it well. Gradually
add the rest of the liquid, stirring all the time, until the paste is the same
consistency as toothpaste.

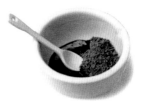

3 Make sure there are no lumps in the paste, then add the drops
of eucalyptus oil and mix well to form a thick lotion.

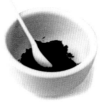

4 Cover the mixture and leave it for about 12 hours to allow the natural
dye to precipitate from the henna.

LEMON AND SUGAR FIXER

You will need this lemon and sugar mixture to fix your design in place so that the active ingredients of the paste can fully penetrate the skin. It is easy to make and should be mixed just before you start painting.

INSTRUCTIONS

1 Strain the lemon juice into the mixing bowl to remove any pips and pulp.

2 Add the sugar and mix well.

3 Wait until the henna paste is dry before applying the lemon and sugar fixer, then use a cotton-wool bud to dab a little of the fixer on to your design, taking care not to rub off the henna paste.

INGREDIENTS

juice of half a lemon or 3 teaspoons concentrated lemon juice

1 teaspoon sugar

EQUIPMENT

fine sieve

mixing bowl

cotton-wool balls or buds (swabs)

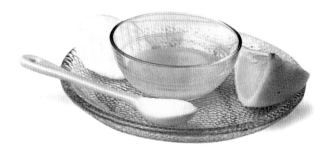

If you are really pushed for time, a quicker alternative recipe for henna paste can be used. Simply mix the lemon juice and sugar solution, as above, and gradually stir in the henna powder. Make sure there are no lumps in the paste and then cover the mixture and leave it overnight. Add the drops of eucalyptus oil the next day, mix it well, and then put the paste in the mehndi cone.

APPLYING HENNA

Your skin is constantly renewing itself and the outer layer – the epidermis – is replaced every three to four weeks, depending on the area of your body. Since henna only penetrates this top layer of skin, and your body regenerates and discards the old skin cells, your henna design will gradually fade away completely. When the henna paste is first removed, the stain it leaves behind will be orange. This gradually darkens over the next two days to a deeper shade of brown. The brighter the initial orange colour, the darker the stain will become. Henna tends to stain a darker shade on the palms of the hands and the soles of feet. Deep staining is linked to the body's internal heat and blood circulation, and as the muscles of our hands and feet are used more than any others, it follows that the stain will be darker in these places. This is the reason why staining is not as dark in areas such as the belly button or arms, but as you wash these areas less frequently, the stain may last just as long.

Bear in mind that skin types vary and this affects the way in which henna is absorbed. The all-important power of the powder is determined by its freshness and quality. For naturally darker skin tones, use a strong, clean mix of henna and avoid using any mixture that is more than three days old as its staining power will be weak.

INSTRUCTIONS

1 Wash and dry the area you wish to paint. A vigorous rub with a towel will remove any deposits that form a barrier between the henna and your skin.

2 Using the henna cone, start to apply your design. Discard the first squeeze of paste as it may be too runny or too thick. Keep squeezing until the paste becomes smooth and easy to work with. Have some damp cotton-wool buds (swabs) and toothpicks ready for wiping away mistakes and tidying up lines. A pin is also useful for clearing out any clogged henna from the top of the cone.

Henna artist extraordinaire, Kiran Sahib, paints the details of a vine.

3 When you have finished painting your design, relax while it dries. You should keep an eye on the henna, making sure it dries evenly and flat rather than shiny, and without cracking. Expect to wait around 10–15 minutes. If you have any leftover paste, keep it covered and use it up within the next three days. Do not store it in the fridge.

4 When the design is dry, apply the lemon and sugar fixer. Dip a cotton-wool bud into the mixture and dab it over the design, but do not use so much that it drips, as this will spread the henna. Reapply 3–4 times to make sure the henna sticks to your skin, replacing the cotton-wool bud regularly so that it doesn't become too saturated. Make sure you are using 100 per cent pure cotton-wool buds, as synthetic ones can shed fibres into the henna paste. After about an hour, the henna paste will begin to turn black, which means it no longer needs the lemon and sugar to keep it moist.

5 Make sure you stay warm. Heat is essential for the henna to penetrate into your skin, so remain indoors by a heater and sip lots of hot drinks. Remember that henna draws heat from the body, so the painted area of your skin will feel colder than the rest of your body. Do not be tempted to use a hairdryer to speed up the drying process. The longer the henna stays wet on your skin, the deeper it will stain.

6 The longer you can keep the henna paste on your skin, the better. Anything between 6 and 12 hours will do the job. To protect your design (and your sheets) in bed, wrap clingfilm around your mehndi. This not only keeps the henna in place, but will add extra heat to encourage the paste to penetrate.

7 To remove the henna, dampen it with a cotton-wool bud dipped in any vegetable oil. This loosens the dried paste so it should wipe away quite easily, and it also helps boost the colour. For stubborn pieces, you may need to gently lift them away with the edge of a butter knife.

Do not panic. The colour you have once the dried henna paste has been removed will darken by almost 50 per cent over the next 24–48 hours. If possible, avoid getting the area wet during this time, or at least for the next 5 hours.

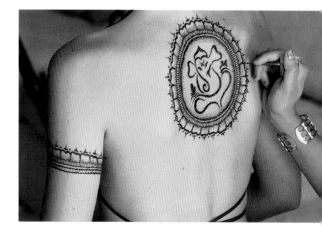

Placement is as important as the design – if necessary, use a ruler to ensure spacing is even.

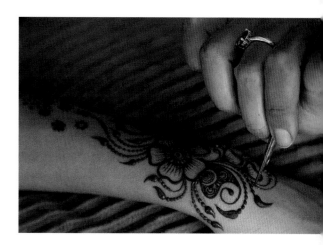

For the greatest impact, consider the point at which the design will stop.

* Make sure you (and the person to be painted) are comfortable. Position yourself so that you have support under the elbow of your drawing hand.

* For intricate hand work, it is best to rest the other person's hands on a table to ensure that they stay perfectly steady throughout painting.

* Never strain your body in an awkward position. It is far easier to stop and reposition yourself than to contort yourself.

* Never touch the skin with the tip of the cone. Aim to lay the henna in lines on top of the skin, not flat against it.

* Learn to control the flow of henna in the cone by squeezing it with just the right amount of pressure. As with any skill, this will come with practice.

USING TRANSFERS

If you don't have a steady hand or feel confident in your artistic abilities, transfers are a foolproof way of achieving complicated, neat outlines of designs without making mistakes. Once the outline has been transferred on to the area of your body you want to decorate, you can then follow with the henna paste in a cone applicator and fill in the pattern.

INSTRUCTIONS

1 Make sure the area of your body to be decorated is positioned correctly and comfortably. For example, if your shoulder is not relaxed when you transfer the outline on to the skin, the resulting pattern may appear to be distorted.

2 If you are using a transfer on a curved area of your body, you may need to make several small scissor cuts around the edges of the transfer so that it will lie flat against your skin.

3 Moisten the transfer and lay it carefully against your skin. Hold it in the centre and gently tap the surrounding areas of the transfer down so that the entire design is pressed flat against your skin. Taking care not to move the transfer, rub it gently several times to remove any air bubbles and make sure the whole sheet has made contact with your skin.

4 Carefully peel off the transfer. The outline of the design should be clearly visible on your skin and you can now use a henna cone to fill in the pattern, taking care to keep the henna paste within the lines of the transferred design.

PAINTING FREEHAND

Good-quality henna paste stains straight away, so practise your designs with a pencil and paper before working on your skin.

INSTRUCTIONS

1 Hold your pencil naturally and practise drawing a row of straight lines next to each other.

2 Next, draw diagonal lines close to each other, and then get more adventurous with swirls and circles. This may seem simple, but it gives you a feel for drawing again – something you may not have done since your school days.

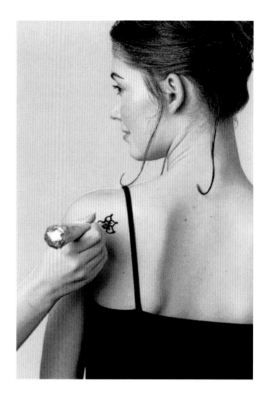

3 Then go over the pencil lines using your henna-filled cone to get the feel of how firmly you need to squeeze it to release the henna paste. There is no right or wrong way to hold a cone, and everyone will hold it slightly differently. The best advice is simply to practise until you discover your own personal style. Once you feel comfortable using the cone, move on to painting your skin.

4 The centre of your palm is a perfect place to begin painting, and you will also get the deepest stain here. A good starting point is a circle, but this can be hard to draw freehand, so use a coin as a guide. Choose a small coin, position it right in the centre of your palm and then press it firmly into your skin for about 10 seconds. When you take the coin away, you will be left with a slight indent which you can carefully trace around with your cone.

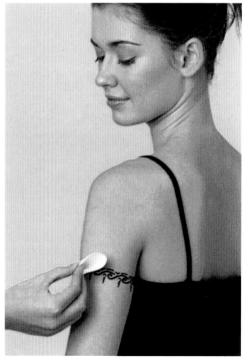

5 As you work, rest the weight of your painting hand on your little finger – this will help balance your hand without touching the design. Position the area you are working on close to your eye level so that you don't need to hunch your back. If you are working from a pattern, place it in front of you.

USING STENCILS

Stencils are made of malleable rubber, which means they can be moulded to fit the shape of any part of your body, and they self-adhesive so they stick to your skin.

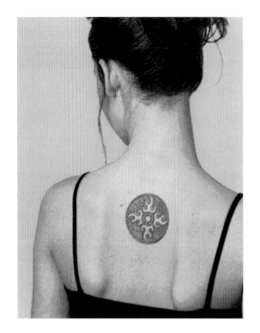
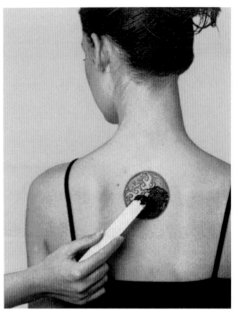
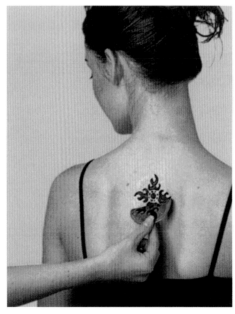
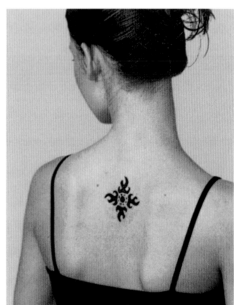

1 Make sure the area of your body you are about to work on is relaxed, then press the stencil on to your skin.

2 Using a spatula, apply the henna paste over the stencil so it seeps into the holes and comes into contact with your skin. Make sure you paint within the stencil so that no henna leaks over the sides.

3 Allow the henna paste to dry, and then use a cotton-wool bud to apply the lemon and sugar fixer on top, as you would over a freehand design.

4 If possible, leave the stencil on overnight. To hold it in place, wrap the area in clingfilm – this will also produce heat that encourages the stain to deepen.

MAINTAINING YOUR MEHNDI DESIGNS

There are a few simple precautions that you can take to help your henna tattoos last for as long as possible. Since henna stains only the top layer of the skin, which is continuously renewing itself, avoid working on any area of your body that will be subject to a lot of friction from your clothes. Do not let your design get wet for at least five hours after removing the mehndi paste. Make sure you moisturize your skin twice a day (but no more), as this will keep it supple and slow down the natural exfoliation process. But allow the body lotion to be fully absorbed into your skin before you dress. Do not scrub the decorated area when bathing, and pat, rather than rub, your skin dry. Always wear a pair of rubber gloves to protect hand designs when washing dishes or clothes. Avoid swimming – especially in chlorinated water – as this dries your skin and quickens the shedding process. Saunas and steam rooms both promote cell regeneration, so avoid these, too. Do not use suntan lotion on the designed area, and do not use any bleach products because these may lighten or even erase your mehndi design.

The first rule of mehndi painting is that each and every design is unique. So because no two paintings are ever the same, try not to be too precise when you copy a pattern, or you won't enjoy the creative experience of self-expression to the full. Allow yourself the freedom to experiment and your skill will soon improve without you having to work too hard at it. Once you have mastered some of the traditional designs, concentrate on developing new mehndi patterns that reflect your own style and personality.

As you create a new design, don't just think about it from an aesthetic point of view; consider, also, how the pattern of henna paste will flow from the cone as you apply it. This means that when you draw the design template, you will need to join together shapes that link in with each other, so the finished henna pattern flows naturally, without any noticeable joins. Bear in mind that boldly painted, strong geometric patterns will look awkward incorporated into the same design as delicate flowery shapes, so within each pattern, choose either a graphic style or a softer look, but don't mix them.

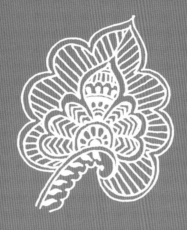

Chapter 4

PATTERNS AND DESIGNS

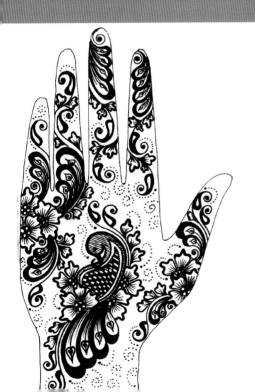
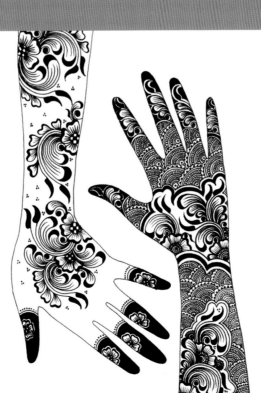
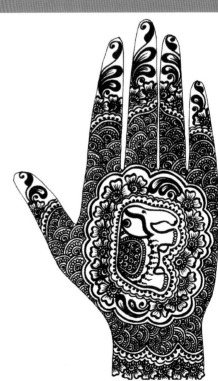

Indivdual Motifs

When you first try your hand at painting with henna, you may find that whole designs are intimidating. But when you consider that most mehndi is based on repetition, all you have to do is to master the basic motifs so that you can build them up to create intricate-looking patterns from very simple beginnings.

1 Draw the outline of a circle using a small coin to guide you (see page 57, step 4), and fill it in.	**2** Balancing your painting hand on your little finger, draw a swirl working outwards from the circle.	**3** Fill in the first shape before moving on to the outline of the next one, and so on.	**4** Repeat this process until you have completed four symmetrical swirls around your original circle.

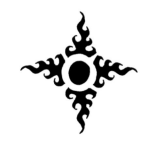

1 Begin by painting a small circle in the centre of your design and fill it in.	**2** Working outwards, paint teardrops spaced evenly around the circle, but not touching it.	**3** Balancing the weight of your painting hand on your little finger, draw a flower around the design.	**4** Carefully add a small dot of henna in the crevice between each of the flower petals.

1 Draw a small dot in the centre, then, with a steady hand, draw a spiral from this point around it.

2 Paint small triangles around the spiral (points outwards) – draw the outline first and then fill it in.

3 Repeat this, filling in the triangles as you go, until they surround the spiral.

4 Next, working outwards from the design, paint a swirly line between each triangle.

 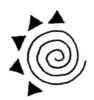 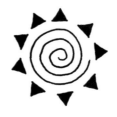 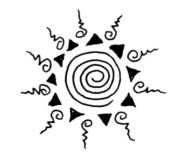

1 Begin with a dot in the middle of the area you want to paint, and then draw a circle around it.

2 Balancing your painting hand on your little finger, paint four teardrop shapes, extending outwards.

3 Make a circle outside the first and fill in the space. Draw heart-shaped petals around the teardrops.

4 Draw S-shaped swirls between the petals, working outwards. Lastly, enhance the design with small dots.

 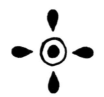 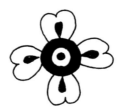 

Traditional Motifs

Build up these traditional mehndi designs on any part of your body.

TIPS

* Start at the centre of a design and work outwards so that you don't run out of space for the rest of the pattern.

* Always draw the outline first, making it slightly thicker than the lines on the inside so that it stands out. Then start filling it in from the top of the design, working downwards.

* Leave a gap of a few millimetres between the lines to allow for the henna to run slightly without spoiling the whole design.

* The thicker and bolder your design, the darker your finished tattoo will be.

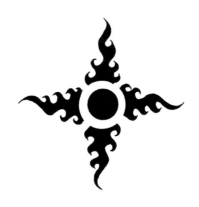
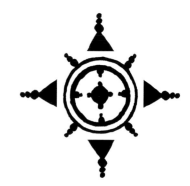
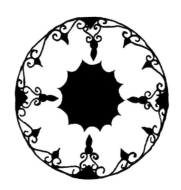
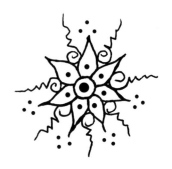
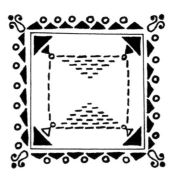
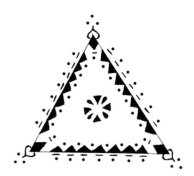

✴ Always start with the basic shape and work from that so the design flows without interruption.

✴ Practise the designs on a piece of paper, then paint over the lines using the cone of henna. When you feel comfortable with this, try doing the same without drawing first.

✴ You'll find you keep a steadier hand if you draw lines towards, rather than away from, your body.

✴ Balance the weight of your painting hand on your little finger to steady it, and take care not to smudge the freshly painted lines.

✴ Keep your body relaxed as you paint. Mehndi designing is time-consuming, so make yourself as comfortable as possible so you enjoy the experience.

✴ The area you are working on should be as close to your eye level as possible so you don't have to strain your neck and shoulders. Mehndi is usually carried out with both people sitting on the floor.

✴ Since a simple S-shaped spiral is the basis of most of these designs, practise it first so you can create your own personal style before moving on to more intricate patterns.

Spirals and Vines

Traditionally linked with happiness, spirals and vines look especially good on wrists and fingers, but can be used on arms and legs, too.

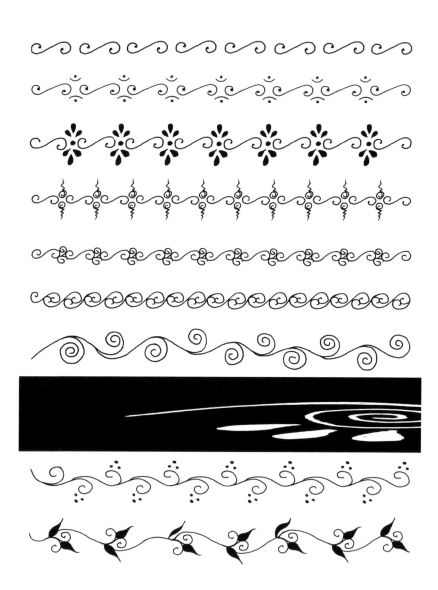

Finger Designs

Fingers are the most expressive part of your body, and accentuating them with intricate henna designs is a very effective way to use mehndi. Painting on fingers can be tricky because of the narrow surface, but working on a small area before moving on to a larger part of the body is a good idea when you are less experienced. The inside of the fingers will stain darker and fade slightly slower than the outside because of the body heat generated from your blood circulation.

* A good starting point is to draw a ring at the base of the finger and extend the design as you become more confident.

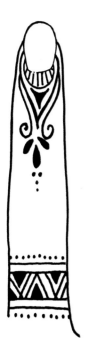 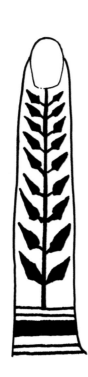 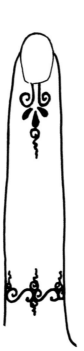 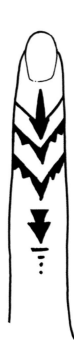 

Wrist and Armbands

These are not traditional places to paint henna, but they have been adopted by Western women as the perfect place to show off a flowing design. The inside of the arm is a preferred spot because the skin there is usually paler and therefore stains a stronger colour than the outside. There is also less body hair to contend with, making it easier to work on.

* To make sure your design doesn't stray off course, place two elastic bands around your wrist or upper arm and use them to mark the boundaries of the area you intend to paint. Another trick is to tape a length of string around your arm to use as a guide to help you paint a perfectly straight line.

* Start by drawing the outlines first and then work in towards the centre.

Hands and Feet

TIPS

* When painting someone's foot, place it on a low stool or table to give you a better angle to work from; it means you won't have to lie on the floor when you're painting around the sides.

* Beware if you have extra-sensitive feet, as scraping off the henna can tickle.

Hands and feet are the places that were traditionally painted with mehndi – they were the only areas that were visible, since the rest of the body had to be covered. Although these patterns may seem complicated, when you look at them carefully you will see that they consist of a series of the individual motifs shown earlier.

While we abuse our feet, women in India decorate theirs with elaborate mehndi and jewellery. One reason for this is that the soles of the feet are believed to be a point of holy contact – the place where a human being and the earth meet. Henna stains the soles of the feet deeply and will be especially dark on the thick skin on the balls of the feet and the heels. Since henna should be left on for several hours, be prepared to stay in one place or have someone carry you around!

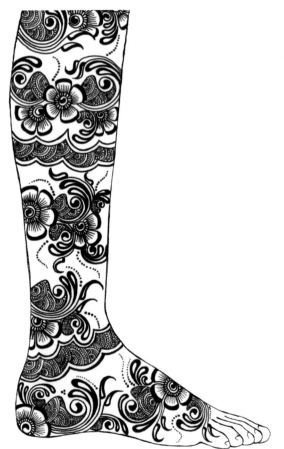

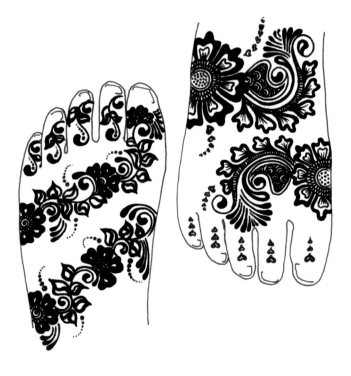

Palms are the perfect place to paint with henna, since they stain more deeply than any other part of the body. Having your hands painted is very pleasurable, since there are hundreds of nerve endings per square centimetre, making them one of the most sensitive parts of your body. It is also therapeutic as it forces you to take time off from your chores while the henna is applied and left to stain the skin. As many women spend a great deal of time with their hands in water, the conditioning henna paste is the perfect antidote for work-worn hands. One reason a bride's hands are painted is because henna softens the skin, which gives her smooth, supple hands for her wedding night.

Line drawings on pages 70–9 by Kiran Sahib – all rights reserved.

* Unless you are looking for an excuse to relax, only have one hand painted at a time. Decorating both means you won't be able to do even the simplest task for at least two hours.

* Be aware that if you extend your design up your arm, the intensity of the colour may vary from that on your hand.

* Start at the centre of your design, then work upwards to paint the fingers.

* If the design begins on the wrist, start there and work upwards and outwards, filling in the design as you go.

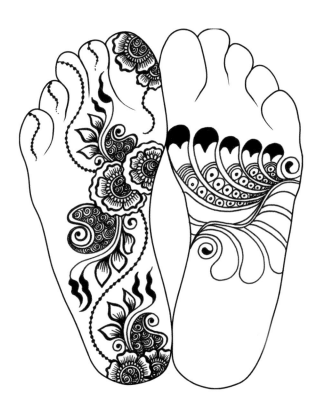

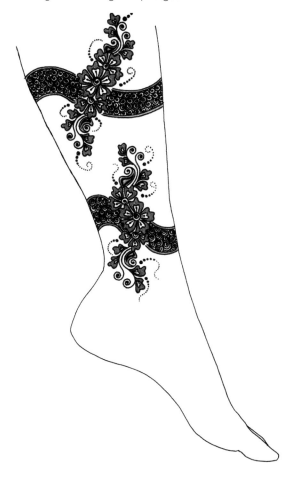

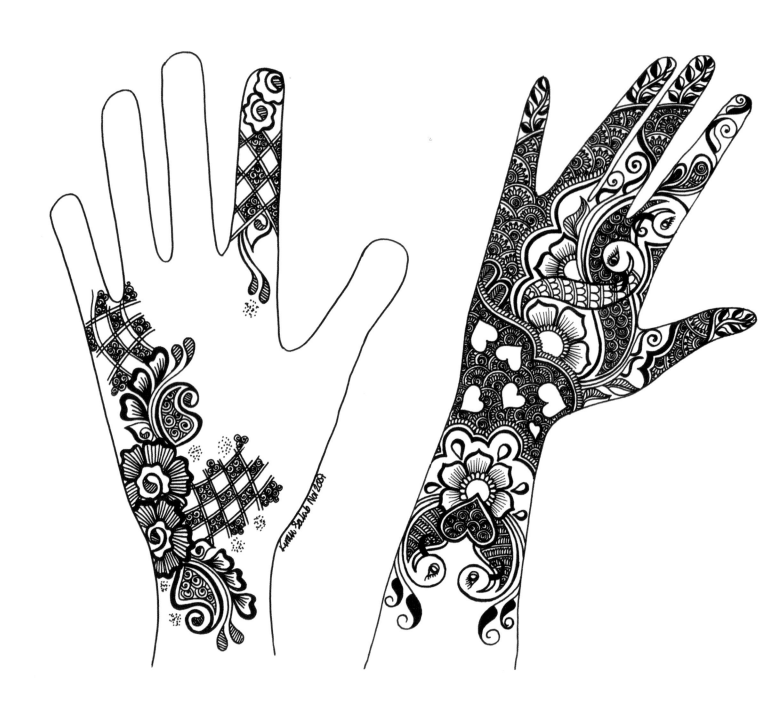

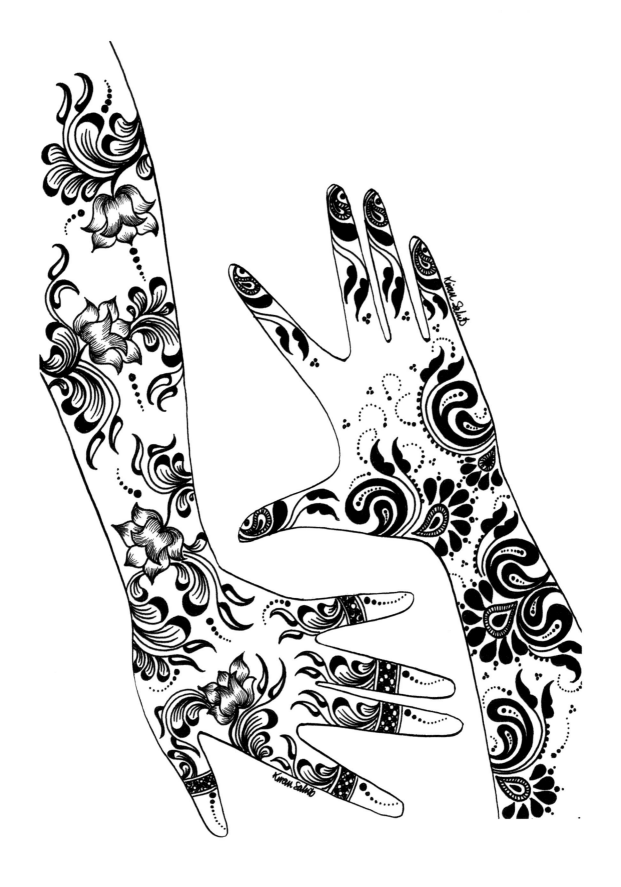

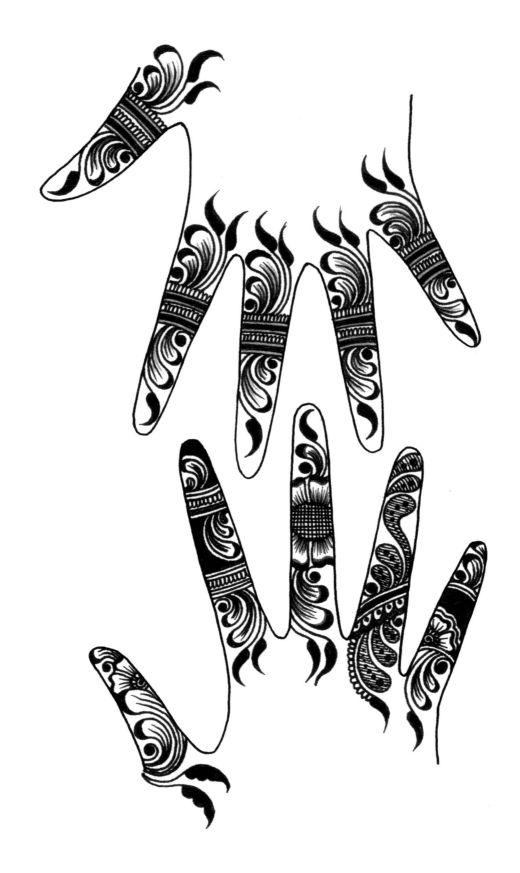

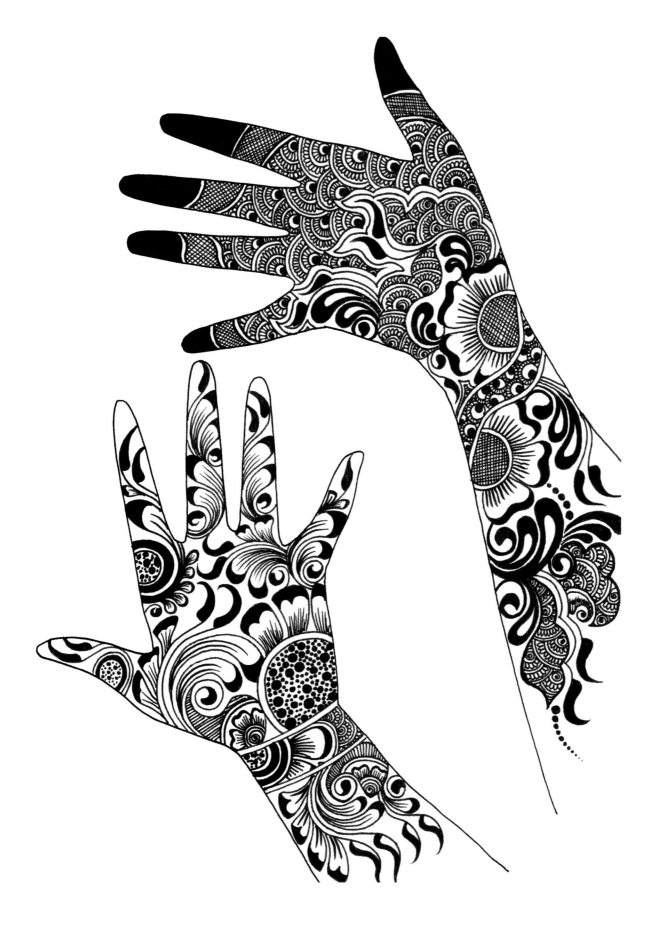

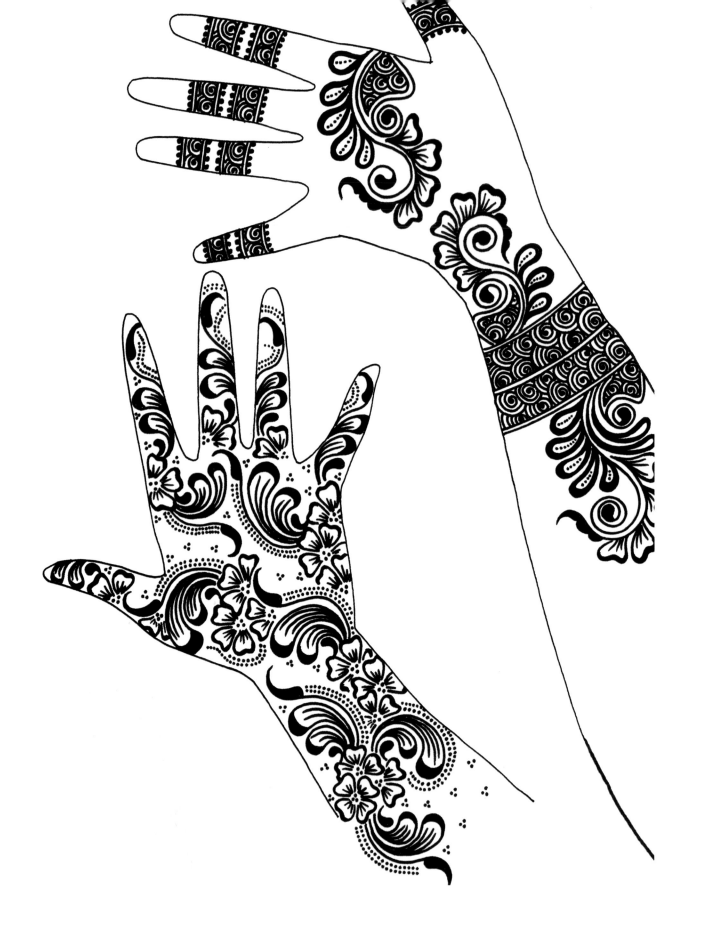

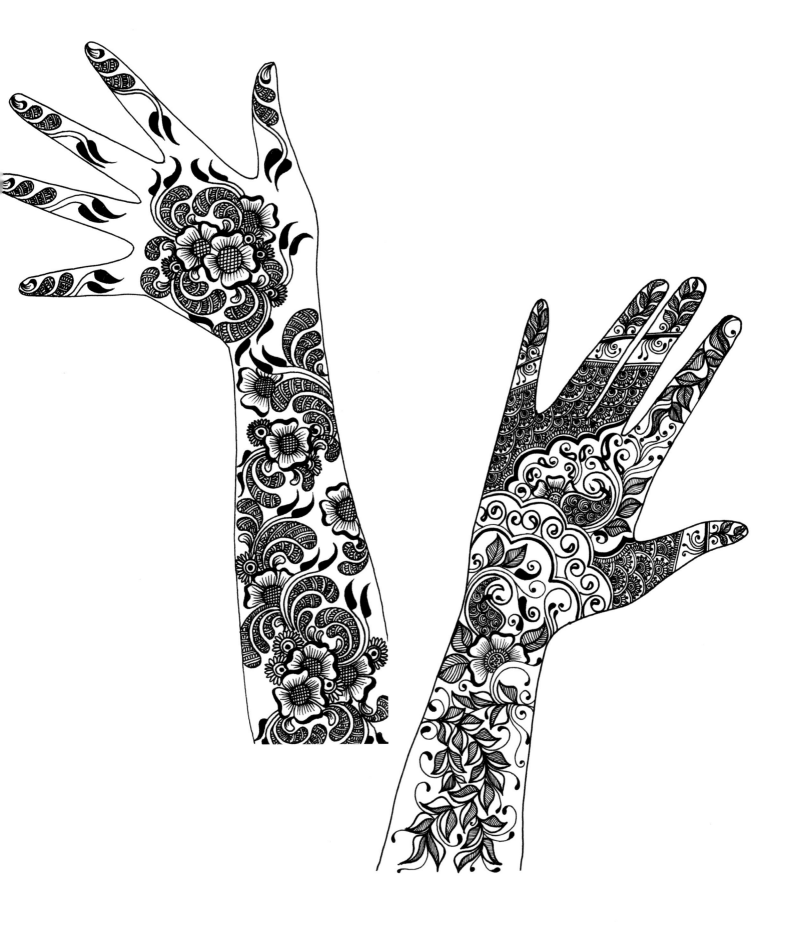

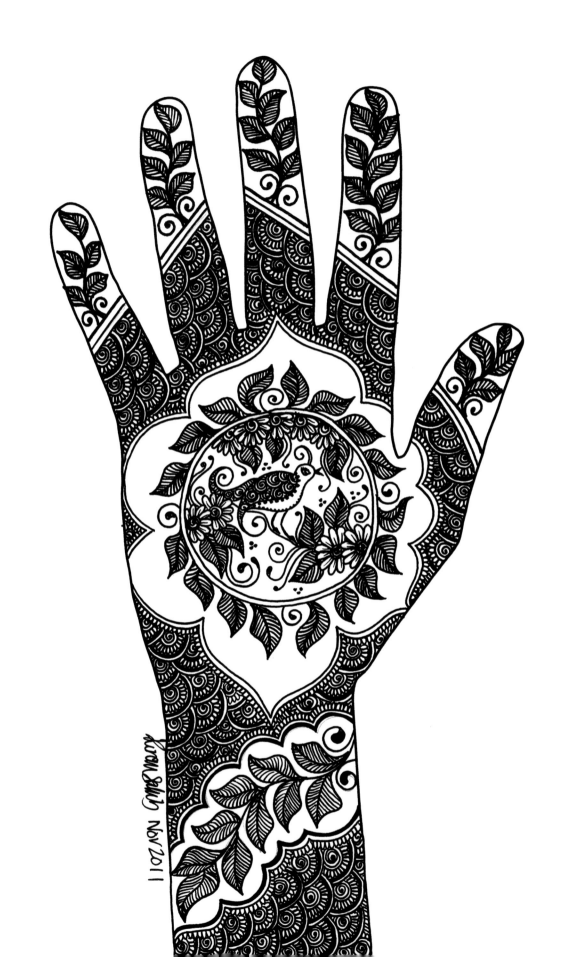

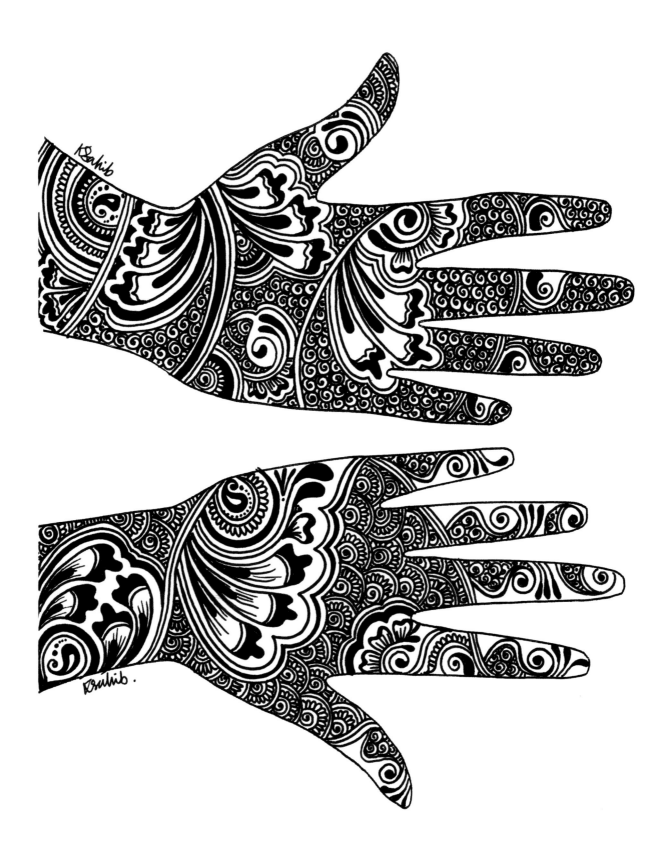

Whether you favour a simple bracelet of interlocking S-shapes, an intricate, embroidery-like wristband or a striking hand motif accented with bindis, the design possibilities of mehndi are truly infinite. Incorporating vines, spirals and dramatic motifs, there is a diverse and stunning collection of henna designs for hands, feet, fingers, wrists, arms and backs. With a wide range of patterns, which vary in degrees of complexity and sources of inspiration, these eye-catching designs represent a two-fold mix of East and West, traditional and contemporary.

The secret with henna tattoos is to master the basic motifs and practise these until you can paint them perfectly and use them to build up your patterns. Each of the following mehndi designs is illustrated with a beautiful photograph and accompanied by clear instructions, so that you can easily duplicate the ideas as well as develop your own original mehndi designs. Elaborate or minimal, dramatic or subtle, these beautiful patterns represent a true East-meets-West experience and, according to tradition, they'll bring you good fortune, too.

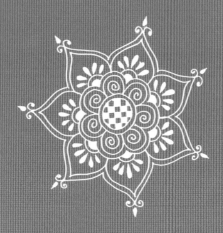

Chapter 5

MEHNDI DESIGNS

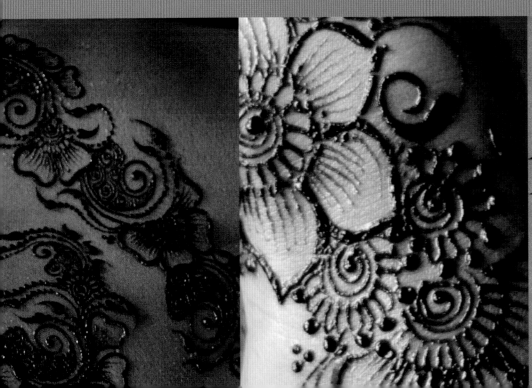

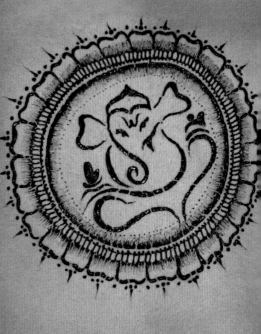

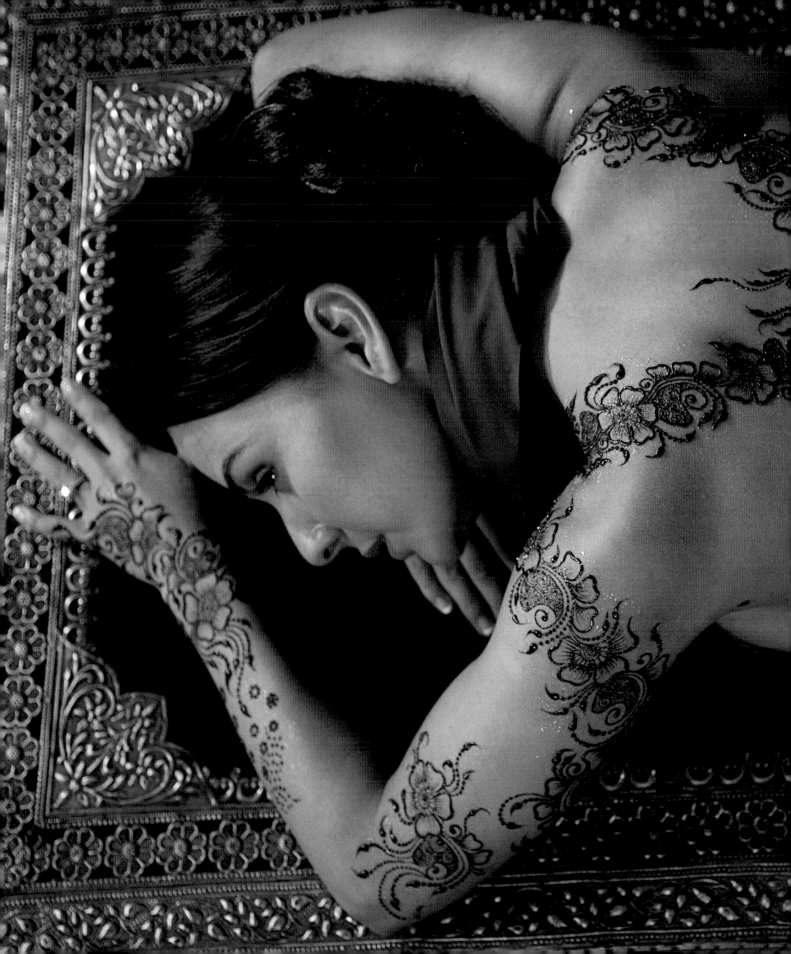

Vine Garland

This design is a collaboration of ideas and styles interpreted and painted beautifully by Kiran Sahib. The blend of Arabic and traditional motifs wrap the model, creating a very sensual vine garland.

METHOD

Start with creating a full six-petalled flower and then attach the paisley motif below. Then go back in to fill in the connecting vines and leaves. By adding flowers with less petals, you can vary the width of the design and enable the overall design to change direction and to flow in an elegant pattern. Be careful to plot out the placement of the interlocking motifs for maximum impact before you begin.

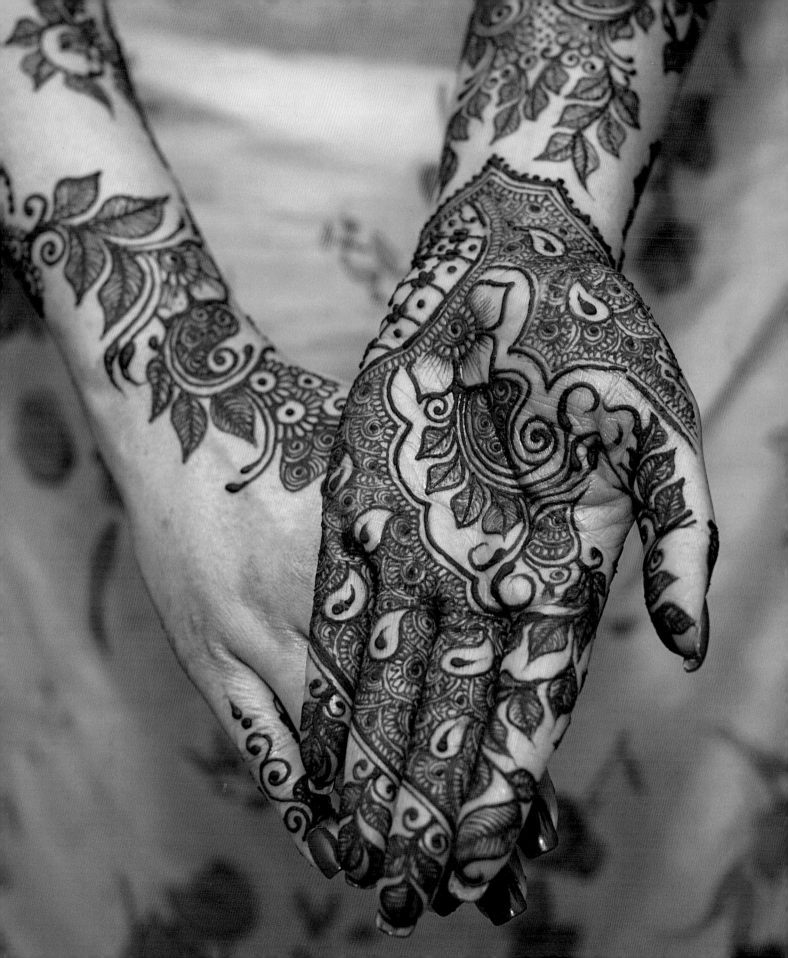

The Kiran Sahib Effect

This hand was painted very effectively by Kiran Sahib. The combination of bold flowers surrounded by intricate filigree makes the area of the hand taht is not painted as important as the area painted. I am a fan of Karan's work because of the patience and time she takes on the detailing.

METHOD

Paint the bold floral vine in the centre of the palm first and then fill in the fine details. Remember to create a balance between the designs, as the effectiveness requires an eye for detail to the parts not painted just as much as the portion you are drawing on. An outcome like the one Kiran attains can only happen with practice, patience and time given to the application. This cannot be rushed and speed cannot play a part in achieving results like these.

Vine Belt

Begin by tracing a diamond shape around the belly button, then enhance the corners with vines or geometric shapes and dots. From the corners at either side of the diamond, extend a vine all the way around the waist to the back.

This design can be used to replace or enhance a belt and is perfect for accentuating a slim waist. Vines are appropriately used here because of their sensual nature. Placing a bindi inside the belly button enhances the effect and catches the eye.

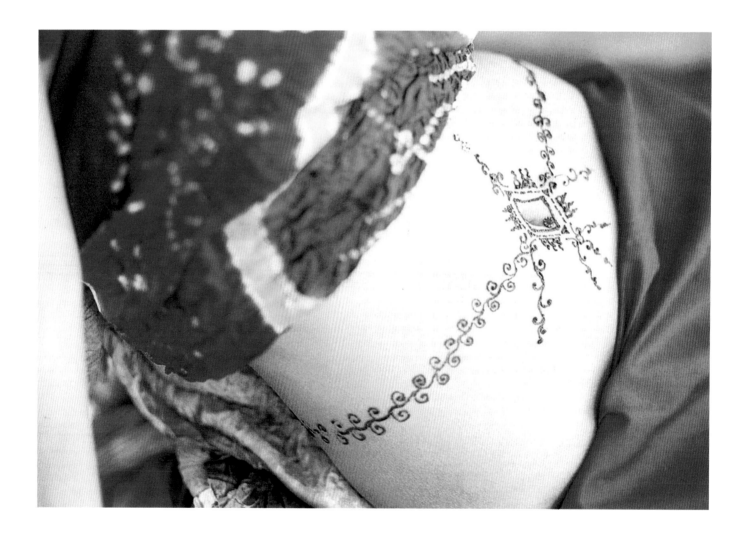

Henna Hand Veil

This vine is used as a replacement for or enhancement of a hand veil. The design is traditionally Moroccan, but is inspired by a piece of Indian jewellery. To make the pattern more elaborate, repeat the design along the fingers.

METHOD

Start by painting a vine bracelet around the wrist, and then extend it along one side of the hand and up the little finger, or any other finger. Try to keep the lines of the vine pattern as straight as possible; if you find this too difficult, then deliberately paint the vine on a curve.

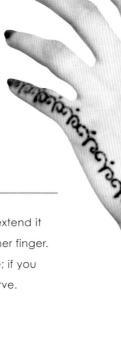

METHOD

Start with a dot in the centre of the palm and build the flower circles and petals systematically around it. Make sure the circles are as clean as possible. Draw small strokes as shading inside the larger, final petal ring. Wrap the design all the way around each finger for the greatest impact.

Lotus Mandala

The lotus is a symbol of purity and used very effectively as a mehndi design. When placed on the palm of a hand, sometimes it is more effective than a full-hand design. The artist, Prabhuti Patel, enhanced this design by adding petals to the tips of the fingers, creating an even more powerful result.

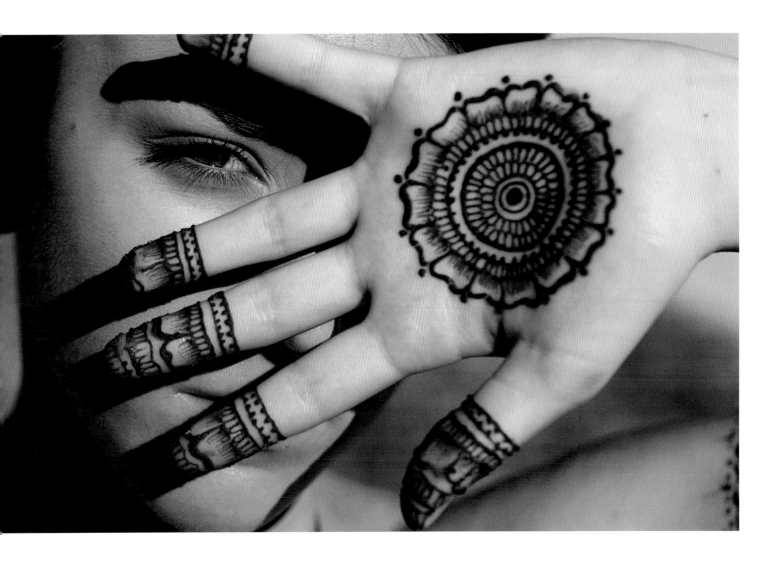

The Om

The Om is the symbol of the deepest and purest voice from within. Wrapped inside a lotus flower, this motif is a representation of deep purity. This is my favorite design and placement for hand painting. I love the interplay of the empty spaces with the decorated.

METHOD

First draw the Om symbol in the centre of the palm, then draw two circles around the Om, adding small dots on the second ring. Draw another circle around this and then add two layers of petals. Enhance the design with petals and dots. Repeat the circles and petals on the wrist to make a bracelet.

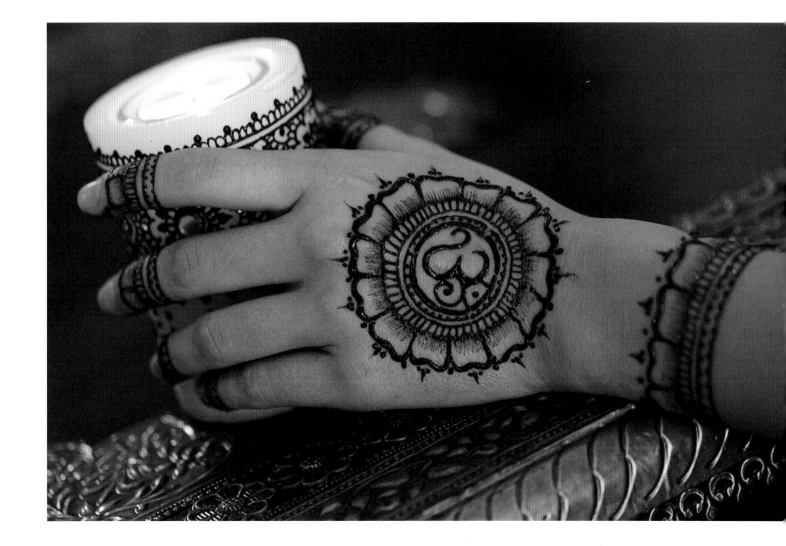

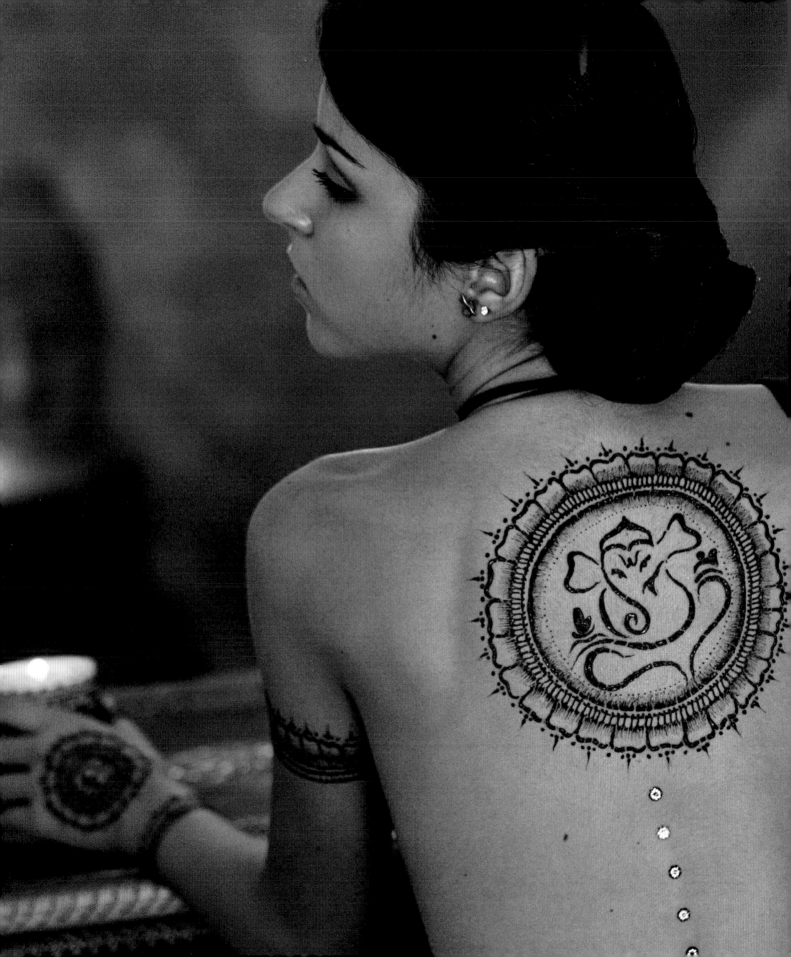

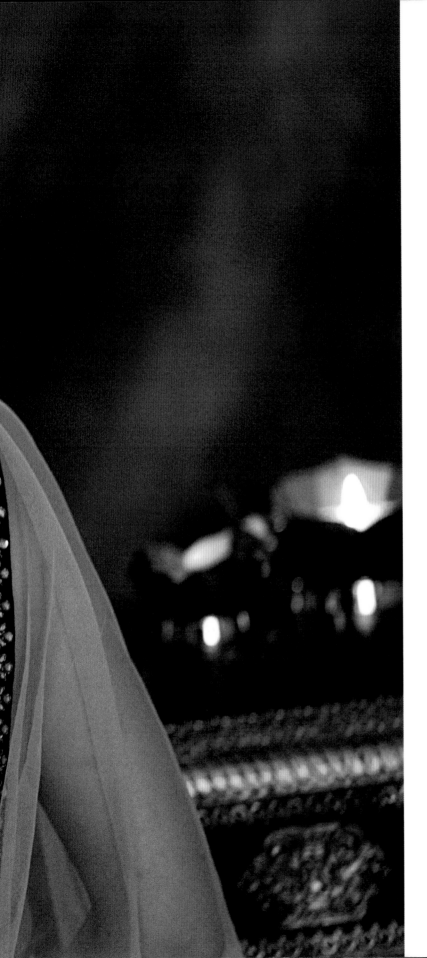

The Ganesha

Ganesha is one of the best-known and most widely worshipped deities in Hinduism. He is popularly worshipped as a remover of obstacles, though traditionally he also places obstacles in the path of those who need to be checked. This design was styled by Sumita Batra and painted by Prabhuti Patel for Ziba Beauty. The Ganesha, surrounded by the lotus, represents the removal of obstacles in your life while the path keeps you pure.

METHOD

If you are not familiar with the image, draw the Ganesha on the body with a pencil first, then go over it with mehndi. Very slowly and carefully create a circle around the Ganesha. Add the shading to the inner circle and then add two more circles with large lotus petals on the outer edge. Enhance with teardrop dots on the outside. You may like to stick on bindis or jewels to accentuate the design.

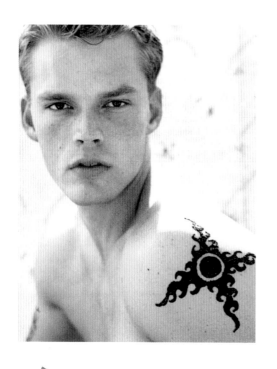

Bold Swirls (male)

This painting of the sun is a popular design for a man's arm or for around a woman's belly button. The sun is symbolic in most cultures and has several different meanings in each one.

METHOD

Begin by drawing a circle and filling it in. Paint four large flames pointing out from the circle in opposite directions, each one comprising several smaller connecting flames, and fill them in. See page 62 for the pattern.

Pure Lotus

Derived from the lotus – the national flower of India – this design represents the inspiration to be pure and upstanding. Being circular in shape, the pattern appears to be continual from all angles.

METHOD

Start with a central circle, then draw three more surrounding circles, spacing them apart as shown in the picture. Fill in the first circle and add swirls inside the third. Place petals around the outermost edge and enhance them with swirls in between the petals. To finish, add a bindi to the centre of the design.

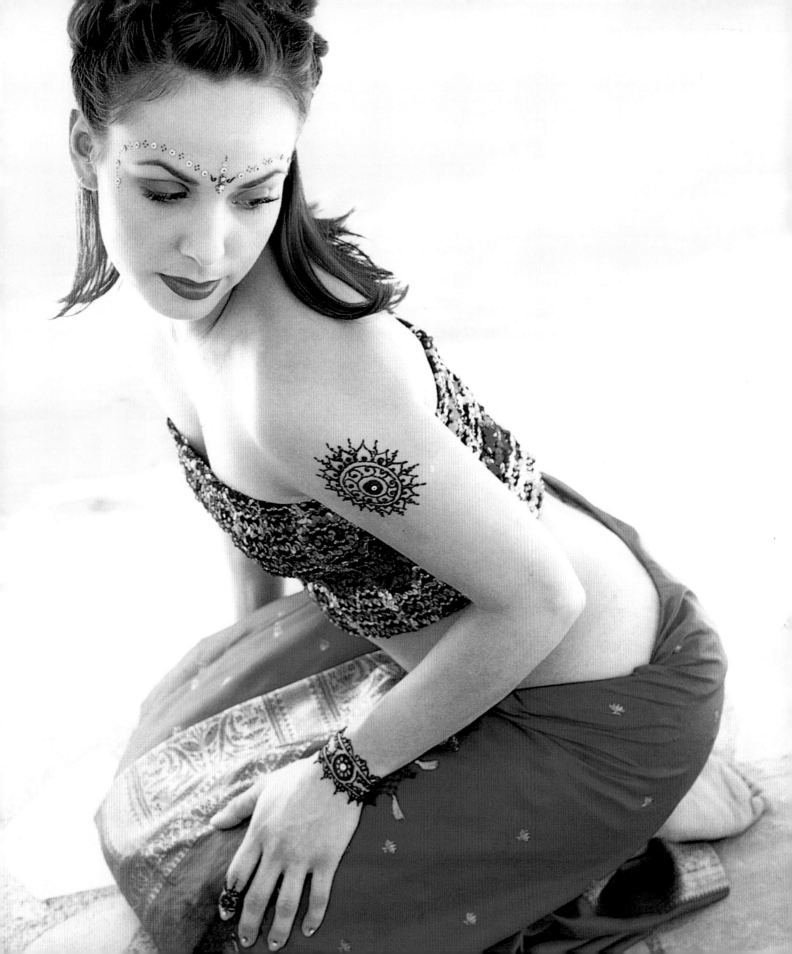

Floral Ring

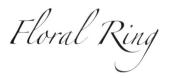

METHOD

Begin with a small flower and build S-shaped vines around the ring to match the bracelet. Enhance the flower by drawing S-shapes on both sides to add thickness and ensure the design looks just like a real ring.

This ring is designed to match the floral bracelet (above). To add to the effect, all the nails have been decorated with bindis. This shows the versatility of body jewels beyond the traditional Indian way of wearing them.

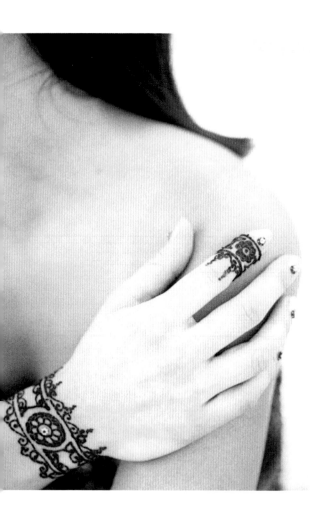

Floral Bracelet

The wrist is a very sensual part of the body and this intricate bracelet that adorns it is a combination of a few simple designs, including S-shaped vines and curves.

METHOD

Start with the outline of a flower in the centre of the wrist, draw a circle around it and fill it in to accentuate the flower. Draw two C-shaped curves on either side of the circle. Extend an S-shaped vine around the wrist from the top of one curve to the top of the other, then make another joining the bases of the curves. Parallel to each of these vines, add a straight line around the wrist, and then paint S-shaped curves on the outer edges of both lines. Between each S-shape, add a swirl to connect them. Lastly, place a bindi in the middle of the flower.

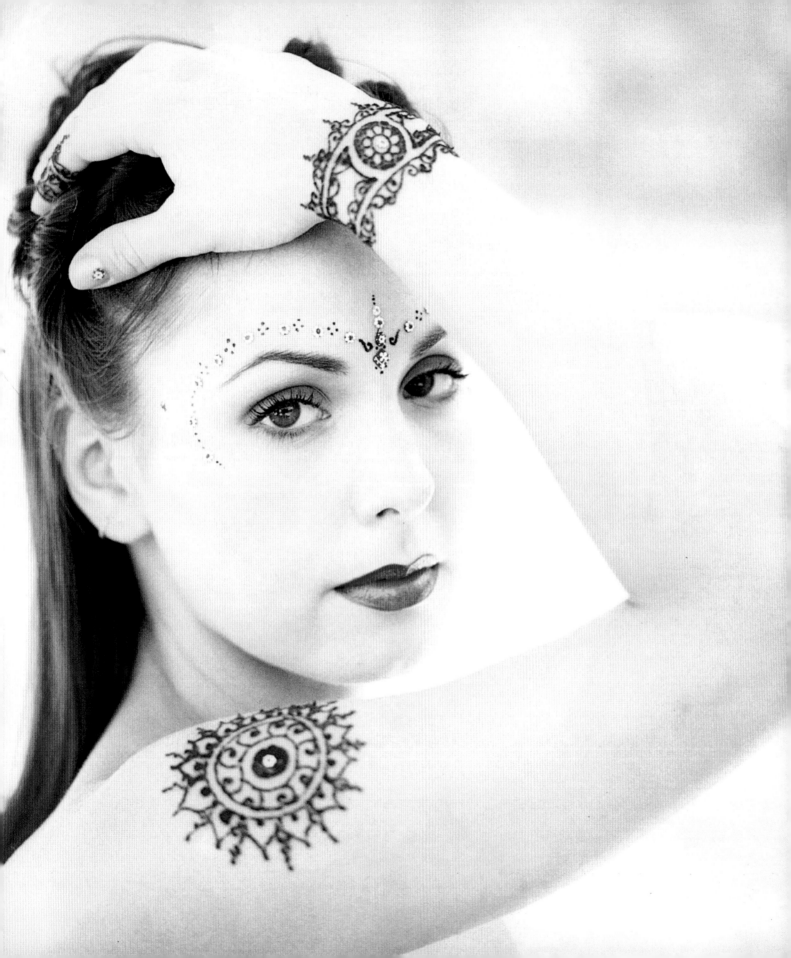

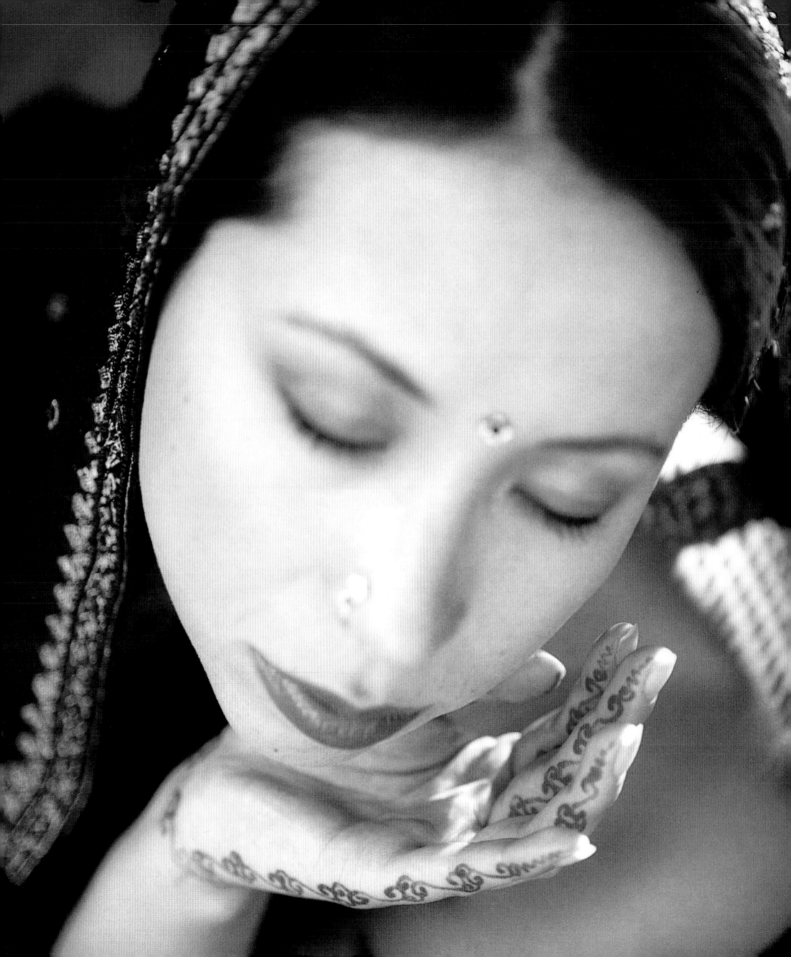

Elegant Delicacy

The key to this subtle design is in carefully placing the pattern along the side of the fingers and outer hand, creating a delicate look.

METHOD

Draw a simple S-shaped vine joined together with small swirls along the outer edge of each finger. Take extra care in positioning the design. Once the henna paste has been washed off, the decoration will take on even more elegance and subtlety.

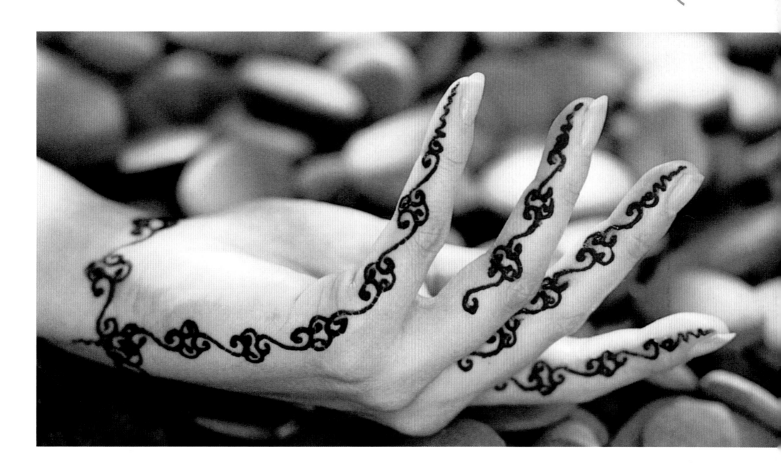

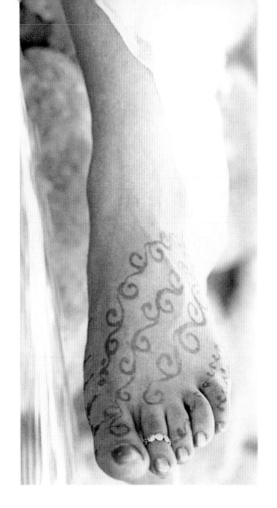

Foot Vine

This design is inspired by a hand veil that has been modified to suit the feet. The subtle S-shaped vine will make any foot look sensual.

METHOD

Work the S-shaped vines across the foot at an angle, beginning at the ankle and finishing at the toes. Work from the inside edge of the foot towards the outer edge, making sure each vine is a little shorter in length than the one before.

METHOD

First draw wide semicircles connected to each other all the way around the ankle, then add half-flowers in each crevice along the top. The bottom part of the design consists of three layers of small connected U-shapes. Add extra layers for a thicker anklet, if you wish. The foot can be enhanced further with a simple pattern.

Mehndi Anklet

Many Indian women cannot afford shoes or choose not to wear them, and instead, enhance their feet with anklets and toe rings. This design is inspired by the traditional anklet worn in India and Pakistan by village women who could not afford fake jewellery for their feet.

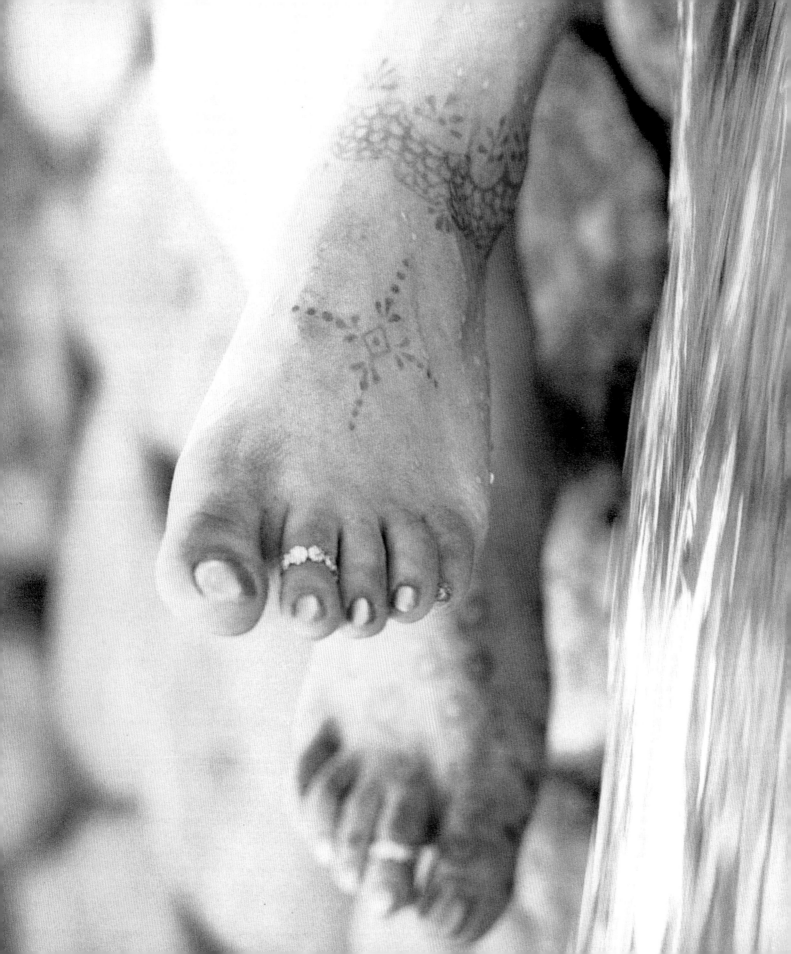

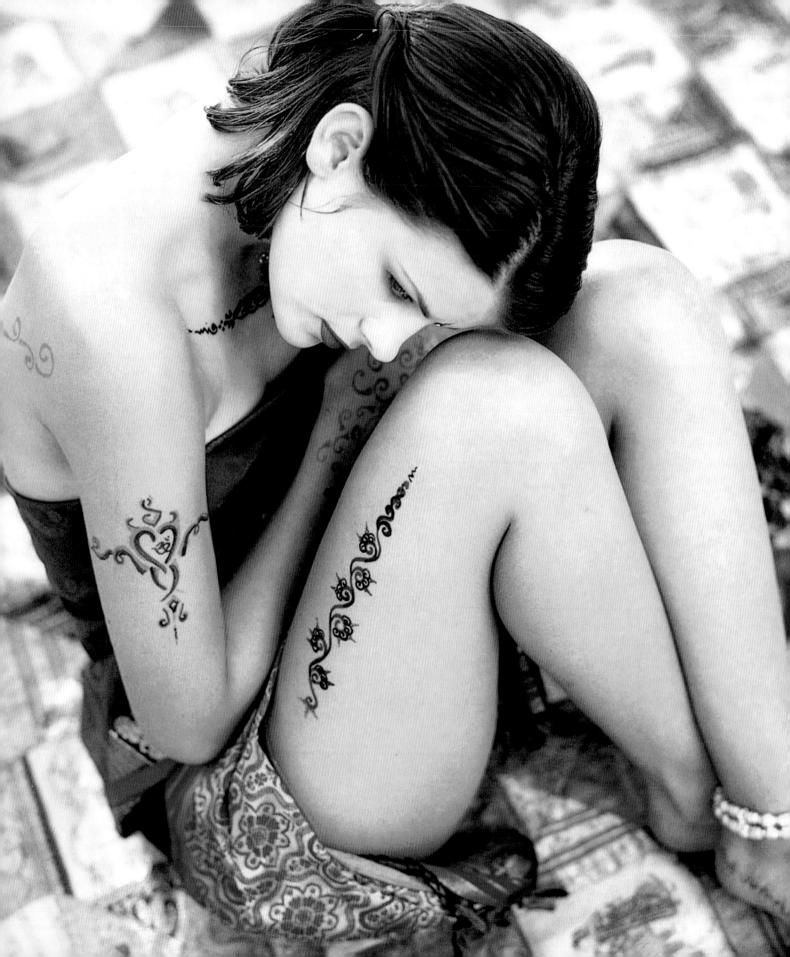

Heart Armband

This armband is a typical accessory-inspired design. The centrepiece is a heart, broken at the top and surrounded by swirls and vines.

METHOD

This design can be drawn using a brush and water-based paints (available from leading make-up manufacturers) for an instant result. Begin by drawing a heart, then accentuate it above and below with swirls. Extend the design outwards and all around the arm with a simple S-shaped vine.

Cosmic Spiral

This elongated design works well on the leg. The linked spiral pattern is repeated to create a sensual tattoo that emphasizes the thigh.

METHOD

Using a thick brush and water-based paints, draw the connecting spiral pattern along the length of the thigh, adding small swirls to each spiral to build up the shape and tapering off to a point at the bottom of the design. See page 68 for the pattern.

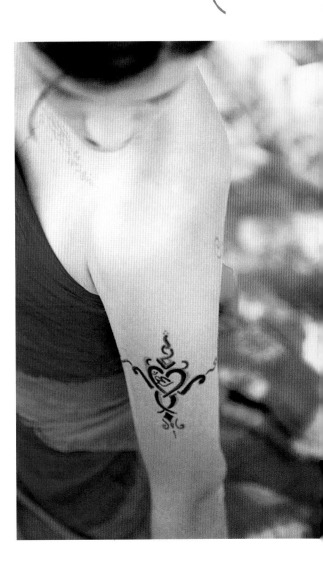

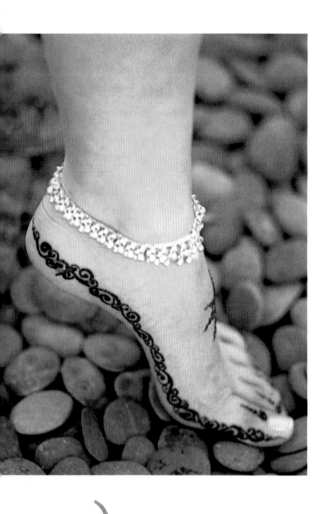

Elegant Delicacy

This foot tattoo shares its inspiration with the similar hand pattern (see page 97). Painting around the edge of the foot brings out the sensual curve of the instep.

METHOD

Rest the foot is as close to eye level as possible, then paint the simple S-shaped vine, starting at the heel and working along the shape of the foot towards the toes.

The Secret Feet

The palms of the hands and the soles of the feet give the deepest shade of stain. This design is a fun surprise for the most patient and creative. Since the stain will be dark, be careful to design enough empty space to get the highest impact between light and dark.

METHOD

Draw a curved vine line and then add leaves on either side. Continue the vine, either connected as offshoots to the main vine line or as separate vines, to follow the curve of the foot in a swirling pattern. Once the vines are complete, add little dot flowers to enhance and accentuate the design.

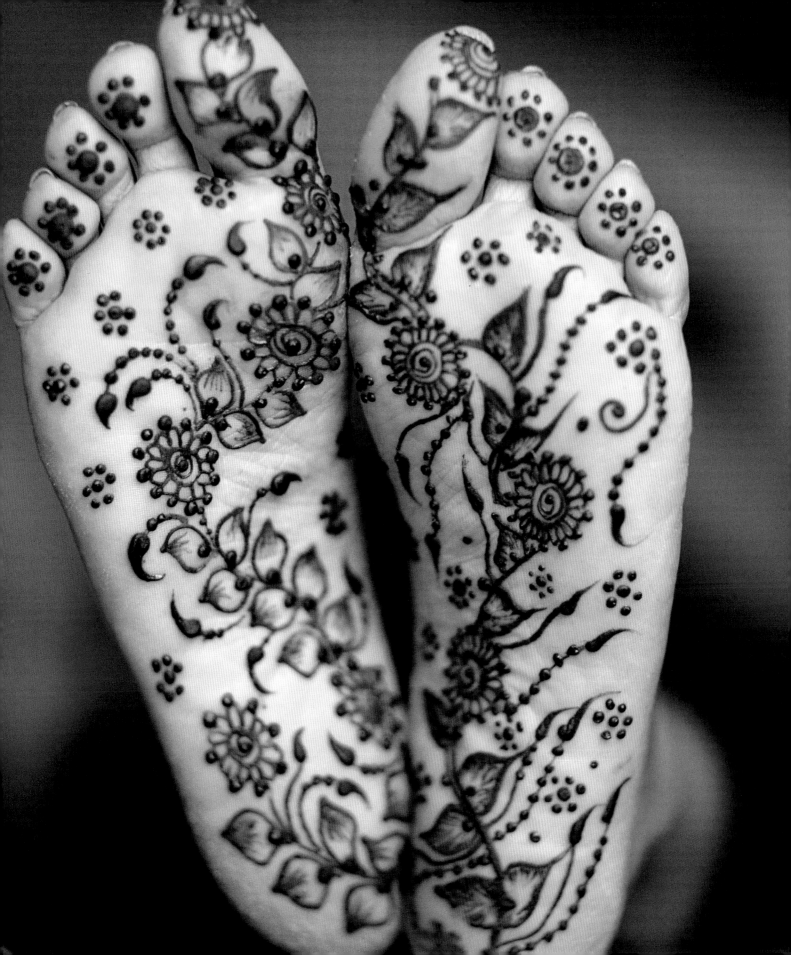

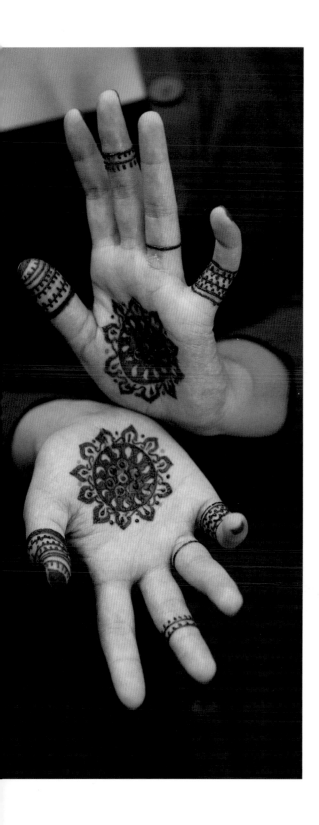

Morrocan Flowers

This design was inspired by Morrocan pottery. The play of negative space with positive space allows for the simplicity of the design to stand out. The fingers were enhanced by simple lines.

METHOD

Start with a dot in the centre of the palm and add a circle. Encircle the central circle with six smaller circles with dots in the centre. Draw a large outer circle. Draw 13 paisley shapes within the circle and fill in the space to leave the paisley shapes white. Draw lotus petals on the outer ring, adding dots between the petals.

Cosmic Armband

This armband is drawn using water-based paints instead of henna. Each S-shaped vine is painted in a different colour and enhanced with a simple vertical line of dots.

METHOD

Draw the connecting S-shaped vine, and add small swirls extending downwards from each spiral. Then draw vertical lines of small dots at evenly spaced intervals around the arm.

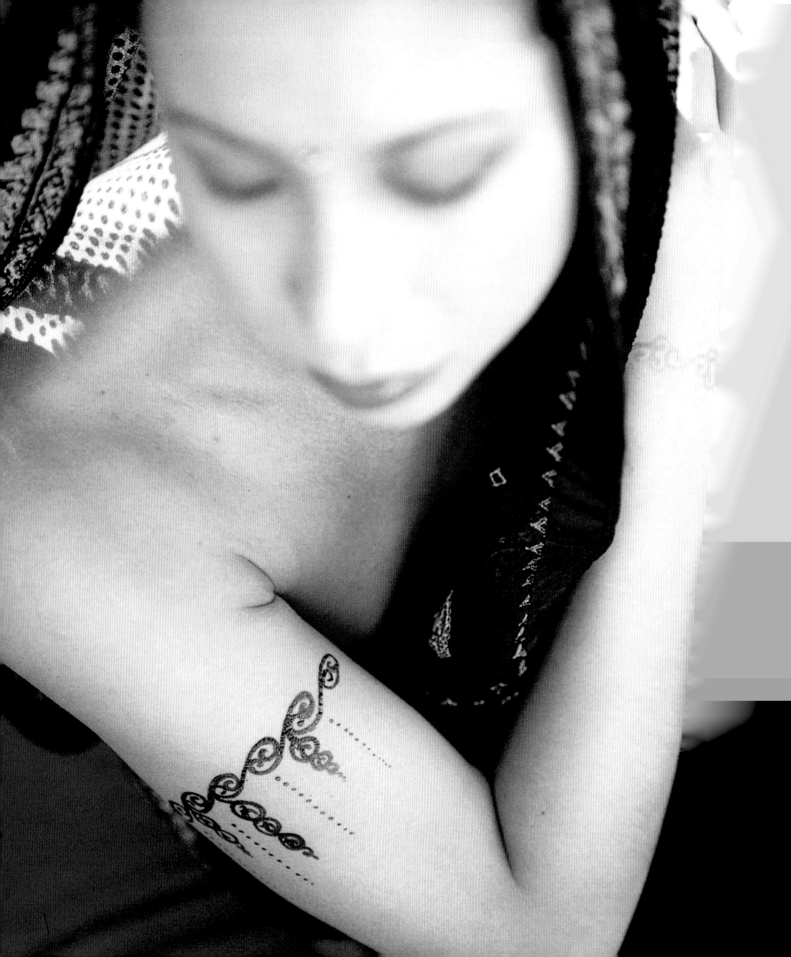

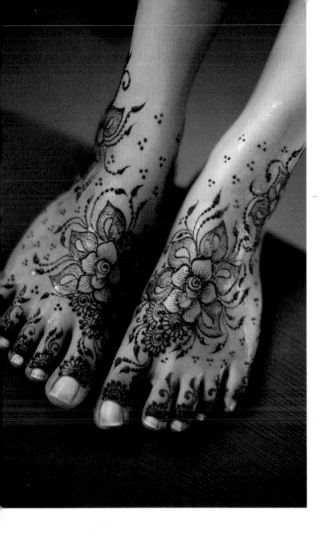

Bridal Hands and Feet

This is a lovely example of Kiran Sahib's detail-oriented work. She is one of the best artists that I have ever had the pleasure of working with. This bridal-work is featured to showcase the detailing and clean lines – especially on the fingers and the toes. This page does not have a method as this is a style of artistry, but it can be used as inspiration for your own work. See also pages 132–9 for more work by individual artists.

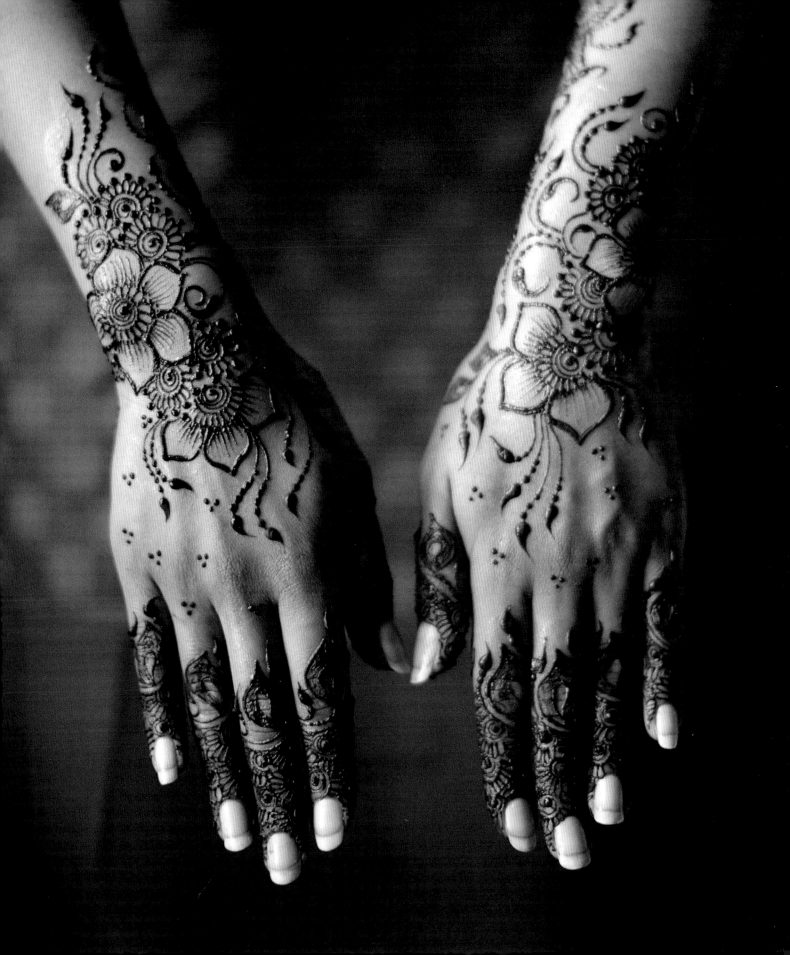

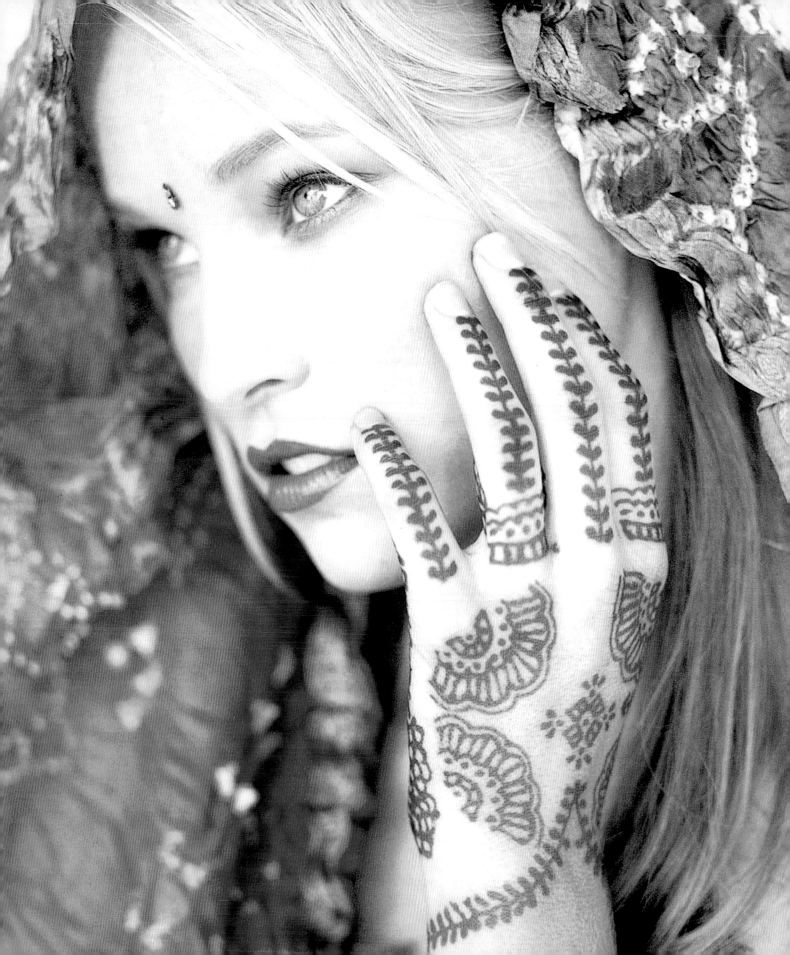

Traditional Indian Design

This is a traditional Indian design, commonly worn by women at weddings. The pattern on the back of the hand is created using the same design four times at different angles. The fingers and wrist are decorated with leaf vines.

METHOD

Copy this design from the picture, beginning at the wrist and finishing with the finger decorations. Concentrate on one area at a time, drawing the outlines first and then filling them in before moving on to the next section (see tips on page 56).

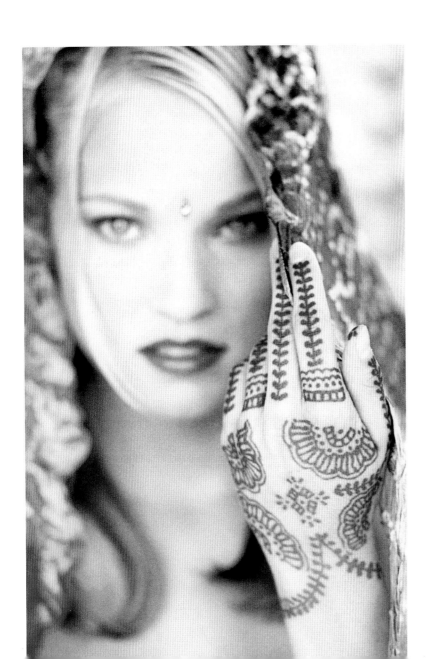

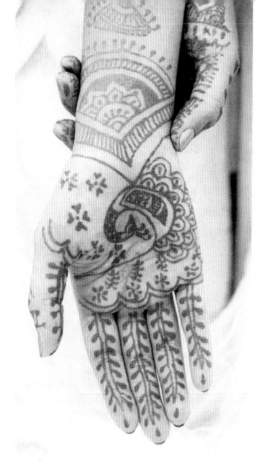

Traditional Peacock

This traditional peacock design is popular at mehndi parties. Typical Indian henna designs show the peacock – a symbol of passion – painted in several different positions and sizes.

METHOD

Closely copy the patterns in the picture, always completing one section before moving on to the next. Start at the wrist and extend the decoration down the arm as far as you like, then build up the pattern on the hand and finish with the fingers.

Moroccan Hand

This symmetrical mehndi pattern is designed to decorate the back of a hand and is inspired by a traditional Moroccan floral pattern.

METHOD

Copy the pattern shown, starting with the central dot. Draw a circle around the dot, add four petals and fill them in. Draw a thick diamond-shaped outline around the whole flower. Next, add semicircles at each crevice and draw three filled-in petals around each semicircle. Finish by decorating the fingers.

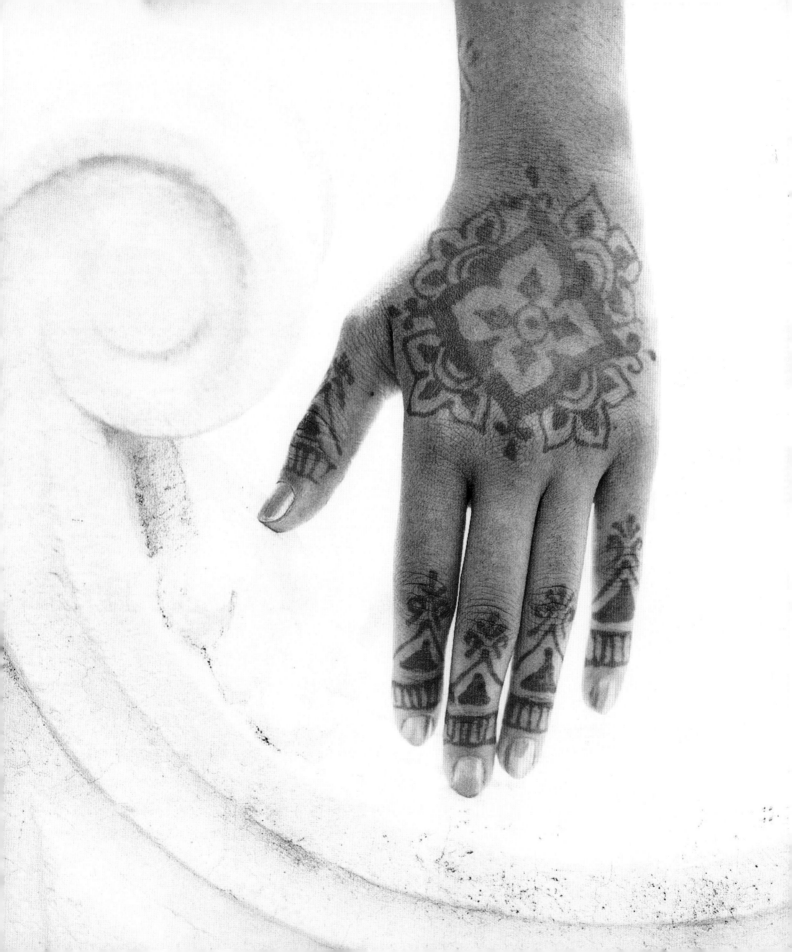

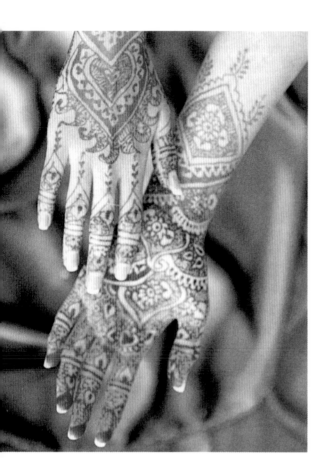

Bridal Hands and Feet

This bridal design is common in India, Pakistan and parts of the Middle East. In a time-consuming process that is perfected only with practice, it is painstakingly applied to one area of the body at a time. To ensure symmetry of design, keep cross-checking between a completed design and the one you are working on.

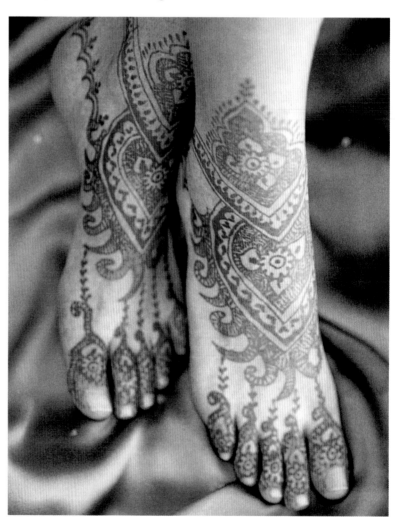

METHOD

The best way to tackle complicated traditional designs like this is to copy the pattern exactly. For the feet, start at the ankle and work towards the toes. For the hands, start at the elbow or wrist and work towards the fingers.

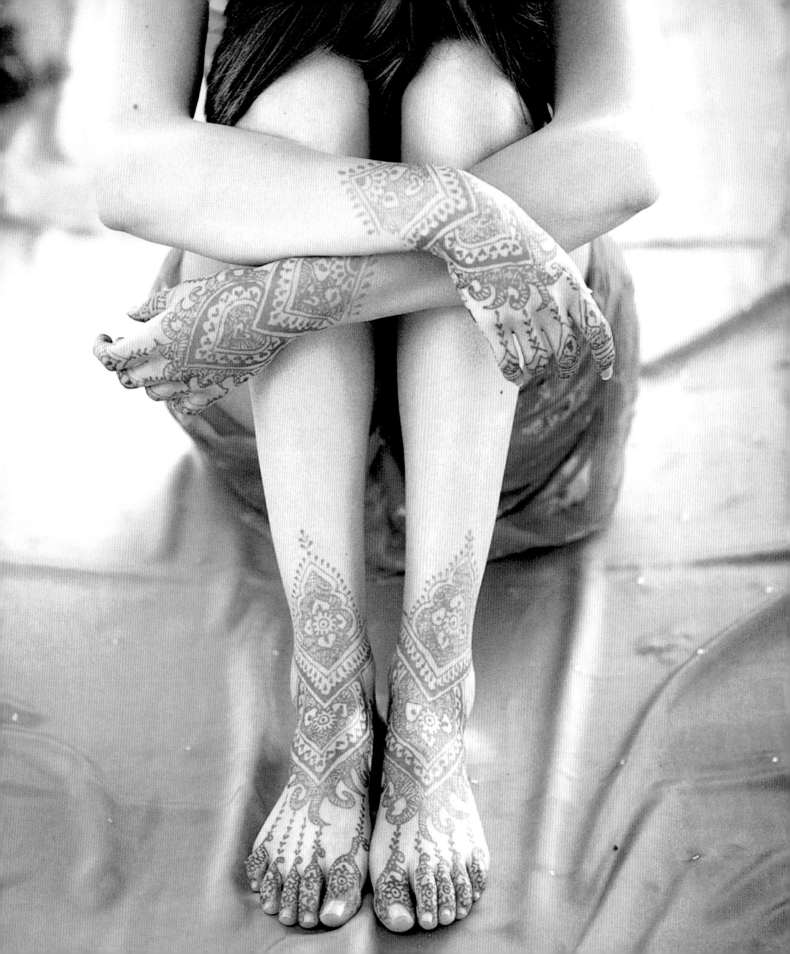

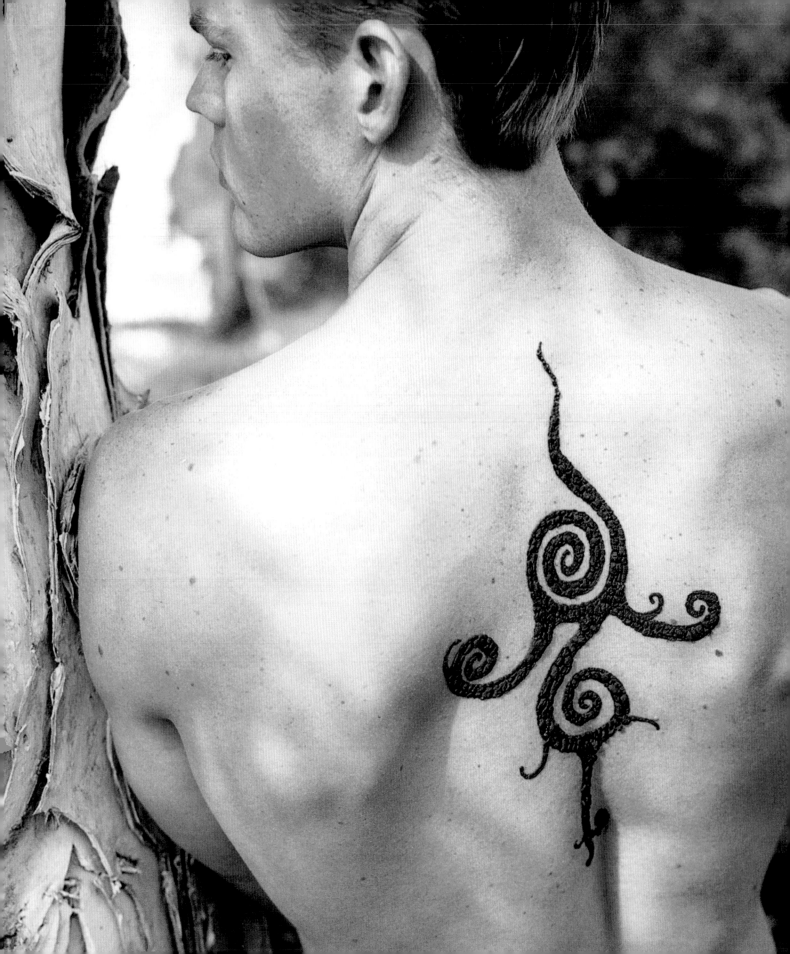

Back Spiral (male)

This is a modified spiral pattern, inspired by the Indian snake design commonly used in mehndi for bindis on the forehead. You can make this as elaborate or as simple as you want.

METHOD

Begin the outline of the central top spiral from a dot in between the shoulder blades, then fill it in thickly. Add the outline of the swirls on either side and fill them in. Next, draw the outline of a second, smaller spiral underneath the first and connect them with a swirl, then fill it in. Lastly, add a downwards swirl from the bottom spiral.

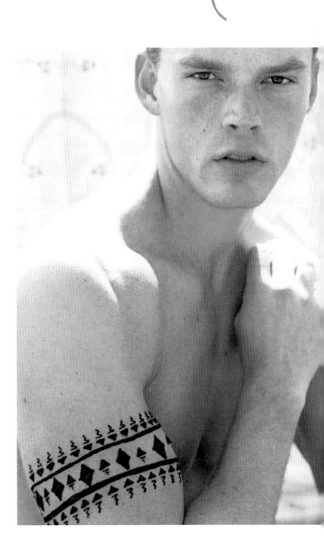

Aztec Armband

This simple armband is inspired by the Aztec patterns of Mexico. The bold shapes make it ideal for men and very easy to draw.

METHOD

First draw a row of diamond shapes all around the arm and fill them in. Draw a single line above and below the design, then paint upside-down triangles along the outside of both lines. Accentuate these triangles with dots or swirls.

Draw a circle at the top of the spine and add the rays of the sun as evenly as possible, extending outwards from the circle. Draw a vine that runs around the sun, and extend it as far as you want across the shoulder blades and down the spine. Lastly, place bindis in the gaps of the vines along the length of the spine.

Solar Mystic

The sun in the centre of this design represents growth and the growing vine is a product of its energy. Bindis running down the length of the spine accentuate the natural pattern of the back's vertebrae.

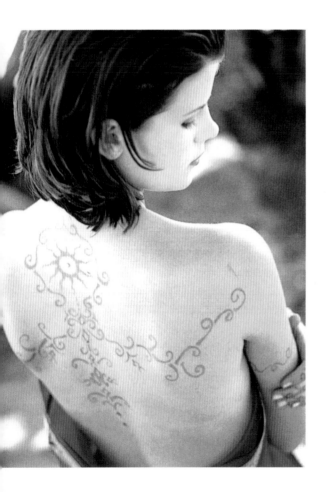

Lotus Vine

This design combines the lotus from India, representing purity, with the vine, which symbolizes strength and perseverance. As an extra touch, the nails have been decorated with bindis.

METHOD

Paint a dot in the centre of the hand and draw a circle around it. Add flower petals all around the circle, then paint another circle around the flower. Fill in the area between the circle and the petals, then repeat the process. Add petals on the outside of the design and enhance them with dots. Extend the design by adding vines to the fingers and around the wrist, working as far up the arm as you wish.

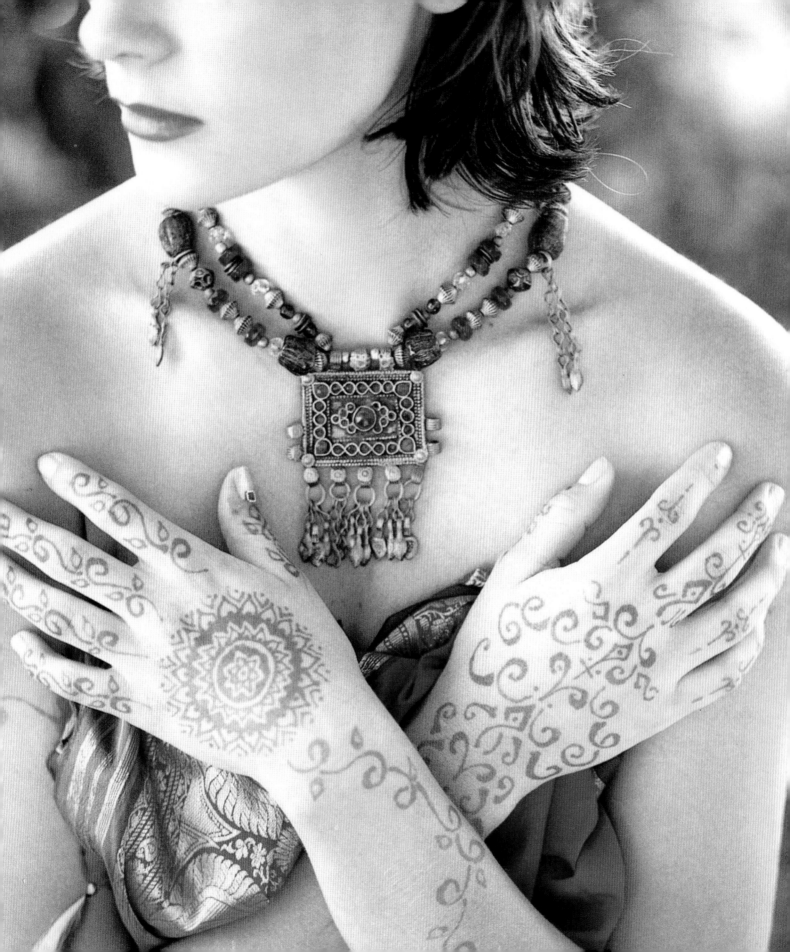

Traditional Indian Vines and Motifs

These designs are commonly drawn by women in India and Pakistan on special mehndi nights. They incorporate the traditional patterns of leaves and flowers, and are easier to achieve than they look.

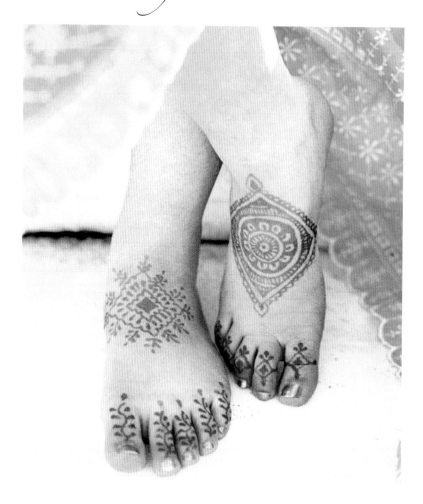

METHOD

The best way to draw these traditional designs is to copy them exactly (see Chapter Four for more ideas). On the hands, first draw two lines to form a large V-shape around the wrists. Working from this point, paint outwards from the centre, adding hearts or leaves on the fingers. For the feet, start at the centre with a dot or diamond, then extend the shape with any design of your choice, or copy this one.

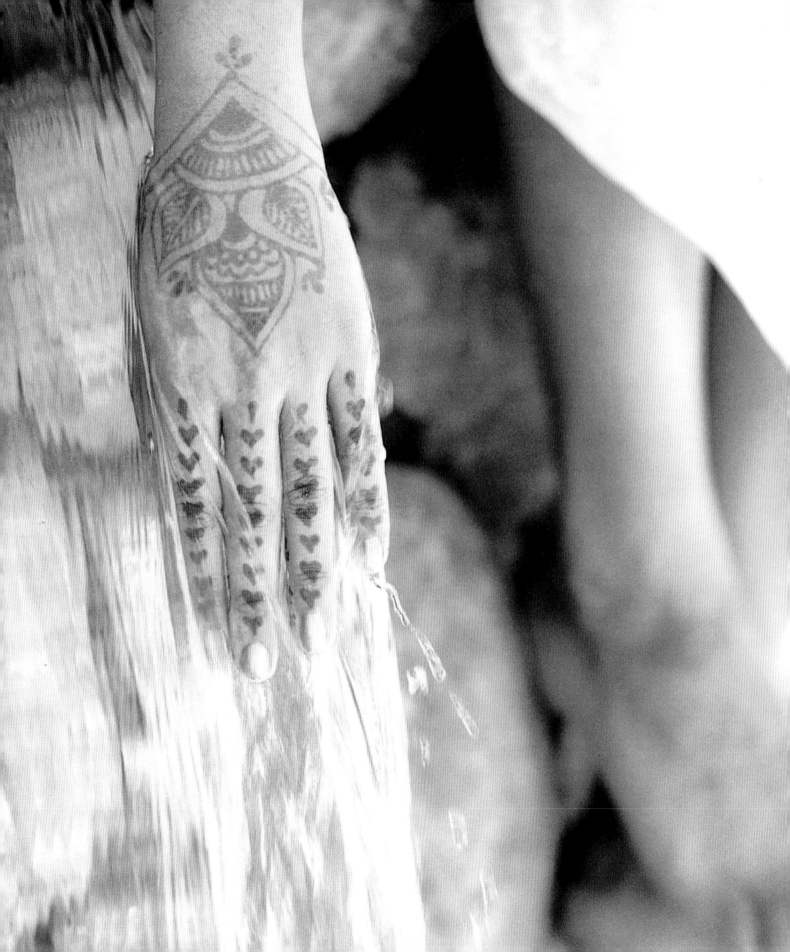

Back Spiral (female)

A more subtle and feminine alternative to the male pattern (see page 115), this spiral design enhances the back and represents countenance.

METHOD

Begin the spiral with a central dot, then add S-shapes around the spiral, enhanced with leaves or dots. Place a bindi in the centre to create a subtle sparkle.

Vine Tips

Inspired by the traditional leaf vine of Indian mehndi, this design is similar to the one worn by Madonna for her 1998 video 'Frozen'.

METHOD

Draw a line tracing the shape of the hand from the wrist to the tip of the thumb and add leaves to both sides. Repeat this on the fingertips, extending it as far as you like.

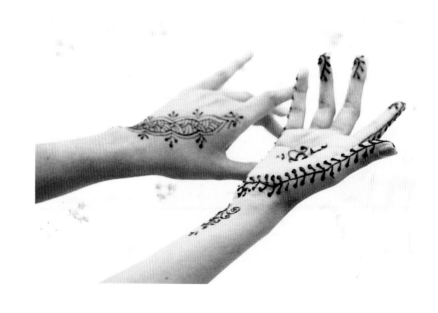

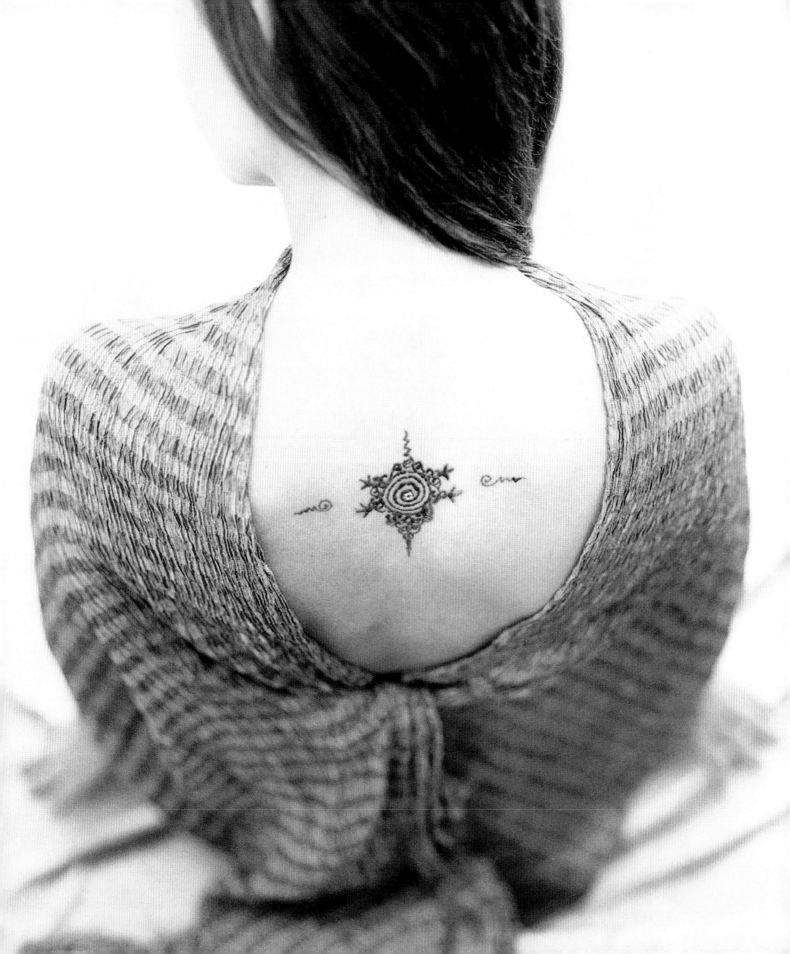

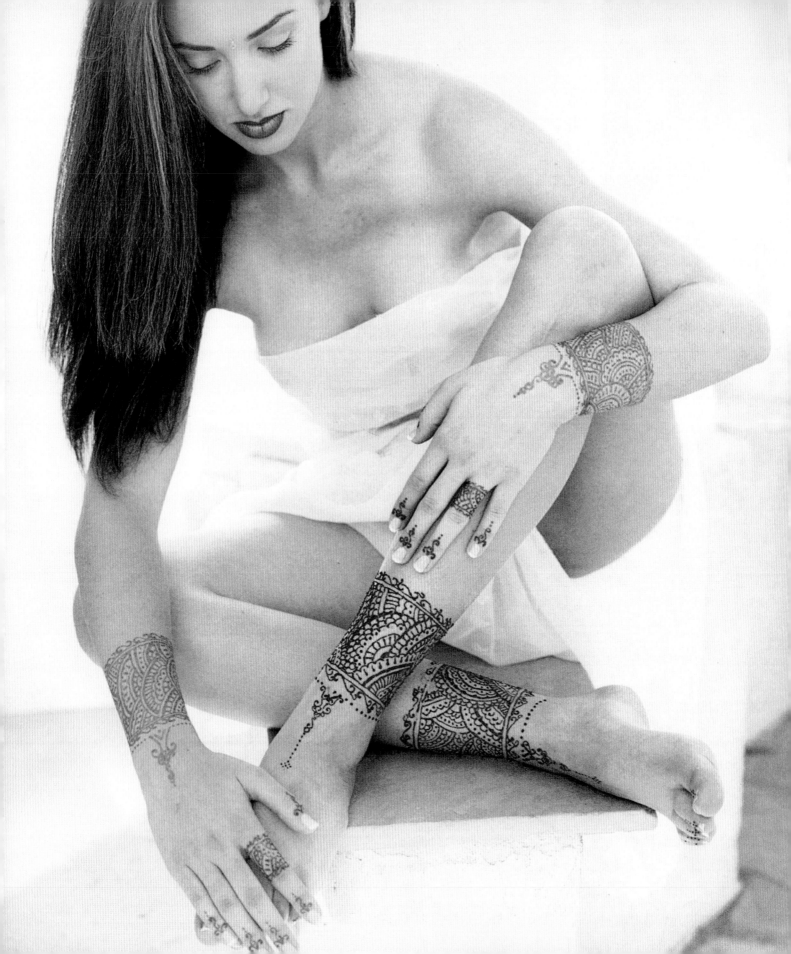

Mehndi Cuff

This design is inspired by the cuff bracelets worn in rural villages in India and Morocco. These chunky pieces of jewellery make a bold statement on delicate wrists and ankles. Although this is a time-consuming design to create, it is worth the effort.

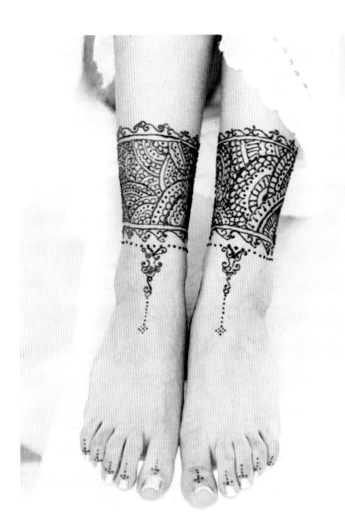

METHOD

Draw a line around the wrist and another above it around the lower arm, leaving enough distance in between to fill in a repetitive design of your choice (see Chapter Four for inspiration). Add an S-shaped vine to the outer edges and extend the design on to the top of the hand. Draw a thick ring on one finger and enhance each of the fingertips with a simple swirl. Repeat this design on the feet, if you wish.

Cuff bracelets make an eye-catching accessory on wrists. Paint your design intricately or simply, depending on the type of effect you wish to create. Use the patterns here for inspiration or create your own unique designs. You can repeat the patterns in miniature around the finger to create a matching ring. To finish, accentuate the whole hand with dots and swirls painted close to the fingertips.

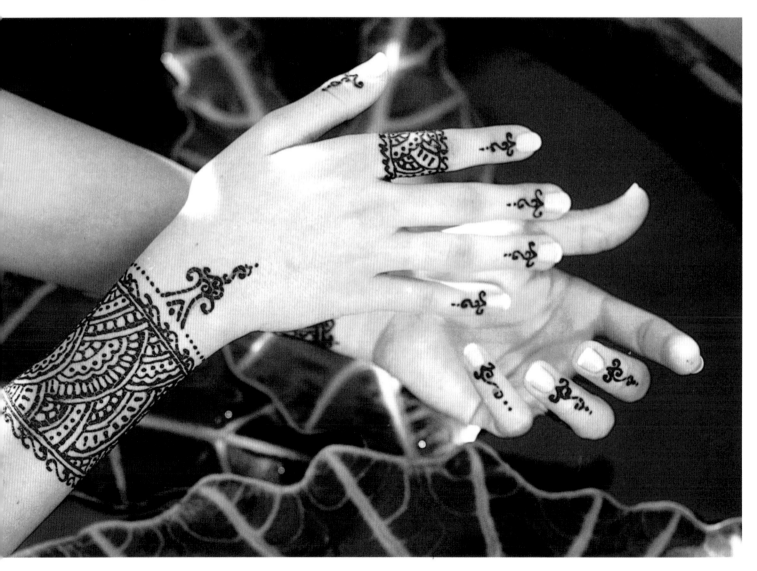

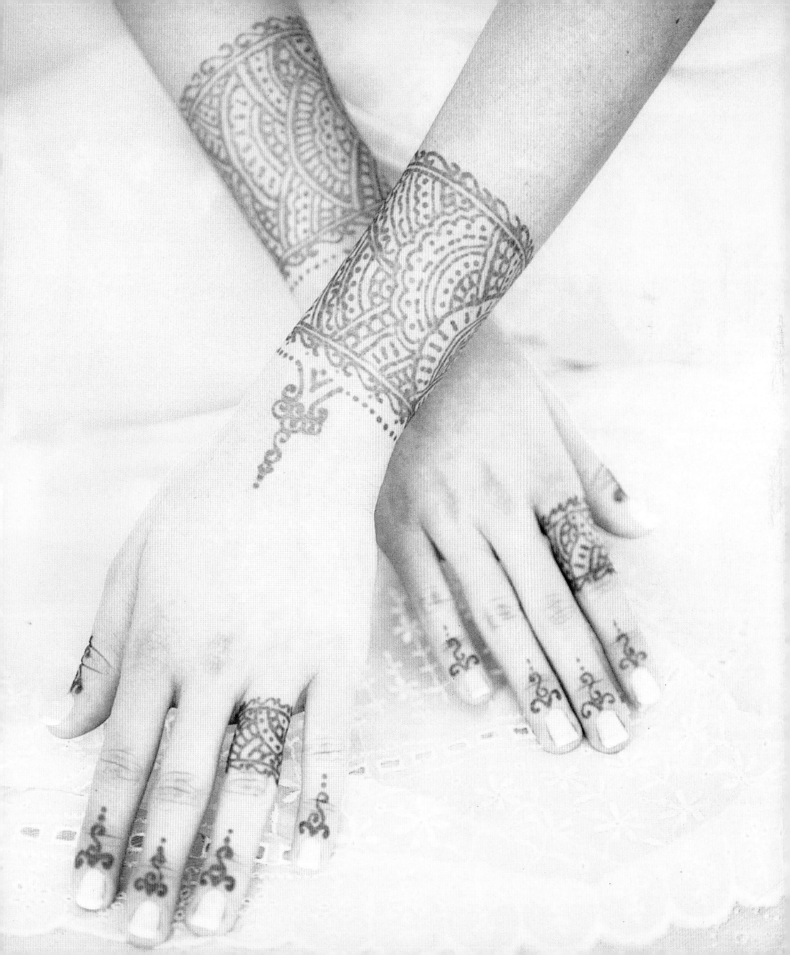

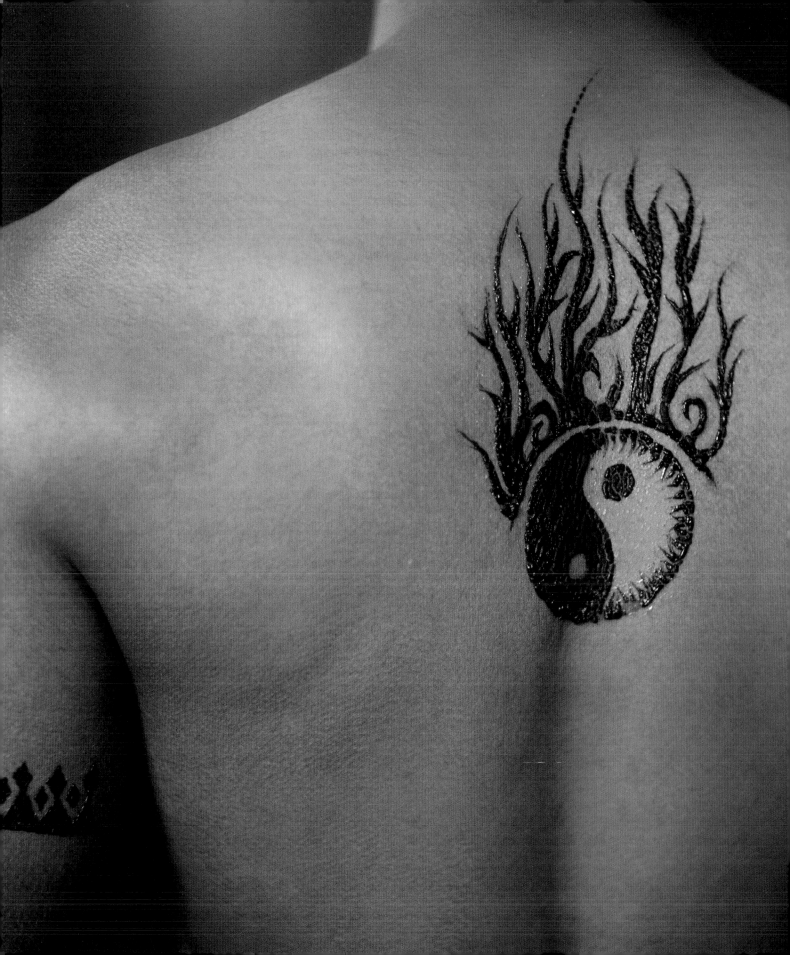

Yin-Yang Sun

Originating from Chinese philosophy, the concept of yin-yang is often referred to in the West as 'yin and yang', which literally means 'shadow and light'. Men are always a challenge to design for but this mehndi shows the strength and power of the sun and the balance of duality represented by the yin-yang symbol.

METHOD

Start by drawing a large circle, and then divide the circle with an S-shape down the middle. Add two small circles on either side centred within the largest area of the pattern. One one side, fill in the area with henna, omitting the circle. On the other side, fill in only the small circle. Make a semi-circle line at the top of the sun, then build flames from the semi-circle to complete design. You can also build the flames around the entire circumference to create a sun effect.

The Paisley

Resembling a twisted teardrop, the kidney-shaped paisley is of Iranian origin, but its Western name derives from the town of Paisley, in central Scotland. In Punjab, India, this pattern is referred to as an 'ambi'. Ambi is derived from the word *amb,* which means mango in Punjabi.

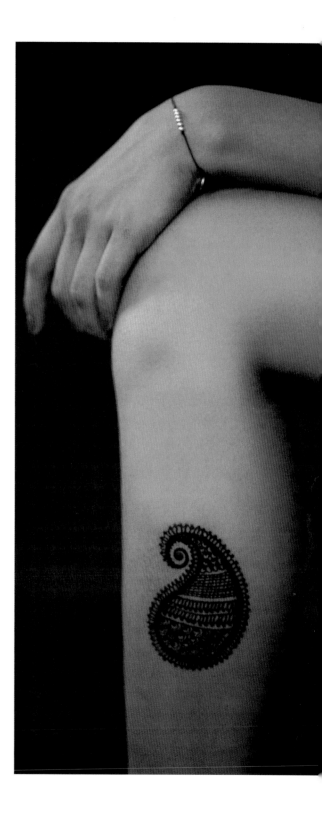

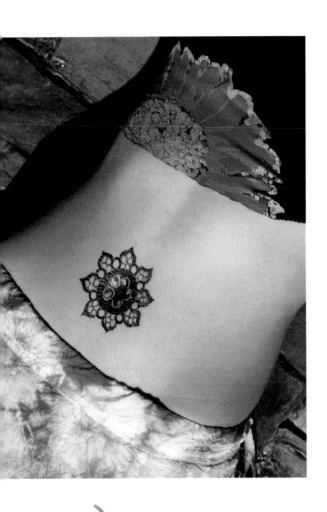

The Belly Enhancer

This is a simple design to enhance and beautify the belly button. It can be done in several different ways and decorated with bindis. Here a series of circles is used to create a lotus-petal design.

Indian Floral Design

This simple Indian mehndi design, based on circles and swirls and enhanced with stick-on bindis, takes on a modern Western look when applied to the shoulder.

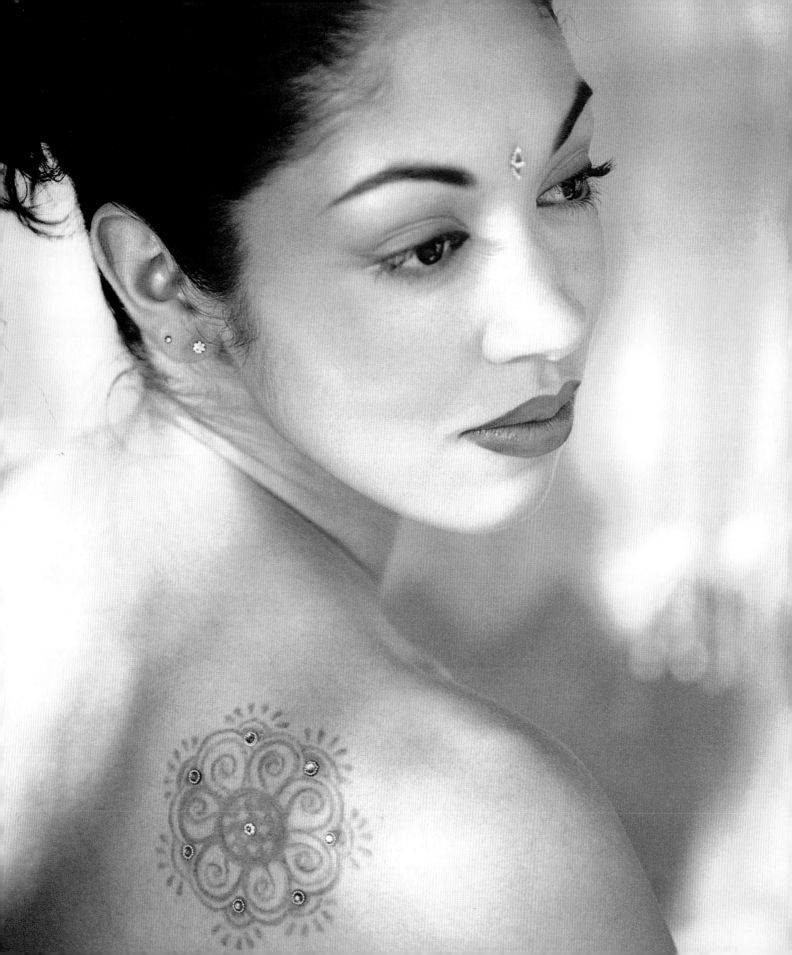

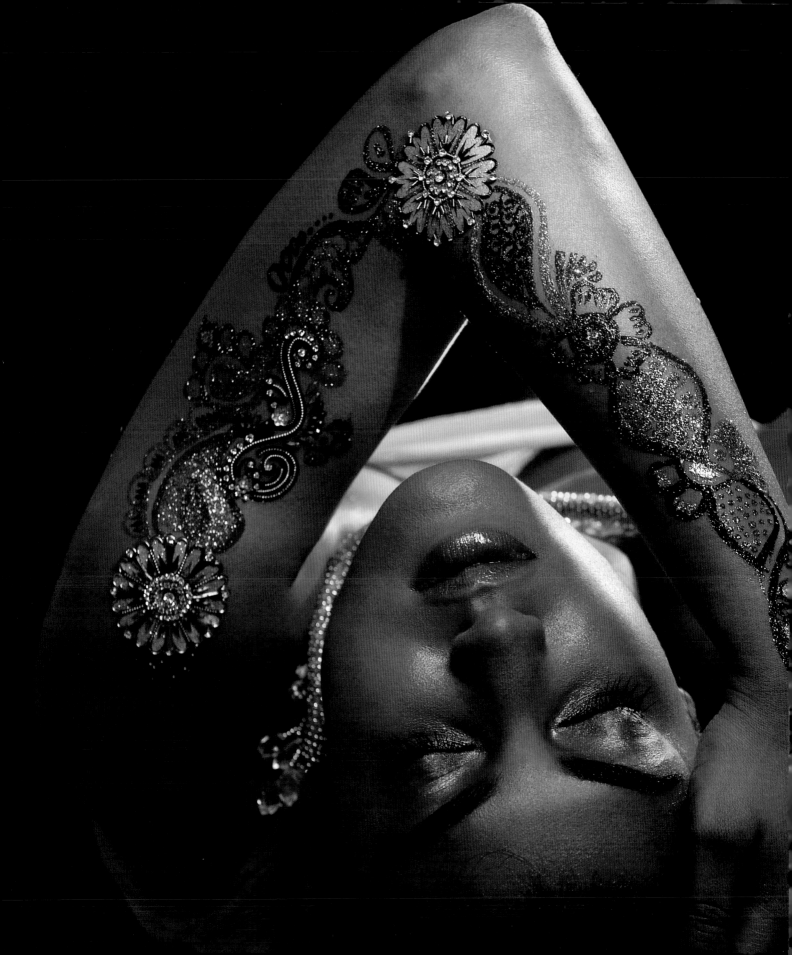

Glitter Designs

When the art of mehndi got discovered by the West, due to its popularity with celebrities and the exposure it received globally from media, one question was asked repeatedly: does it come in colour? I started to experiment with options that could enhance mehndi with colour and formulated a special medical adhesive that is water-resistant. To it I added 24 different shades of extra-fine glitter and today I am able to create beautiful three-dimensional body art that can last up to three days even with exposure to water.

Sumita's glitter designs (opposite and below) use mehndi techniques with colourful glitter formulas to create vibrant works of art.

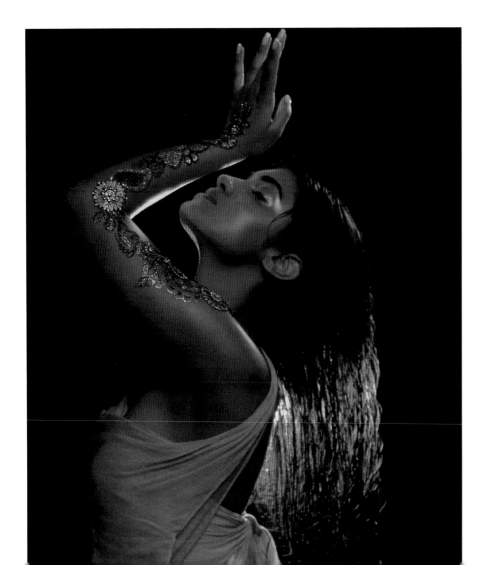

Inspirations

The designs on the following pages are shown here to provide inspiration for your imagination. Mehndi is a highly personal and creative experience, so I encourage you to find your own style and expression. You may look at the positioning of the design elements, the combination of motifs or individual patterns to come up with your own ideas. You may prefer to work in a medium outside henna – for example, by using body paints, cosmetic pencils or stick-on crystals or bindis worked into encrusted, ornate pieces of body art – or a combination!

The cuff (right) is a very popular mehndi request for bridesmaids. This design incorporates paisley with geometric designs. A star, symbolic of divinity and hope, is worked on the hand. Photograph by Yogi Patel – Global Photography, henna by Heta Patel, styling by Sumita Batra, makeup by Oscar Naranjo.

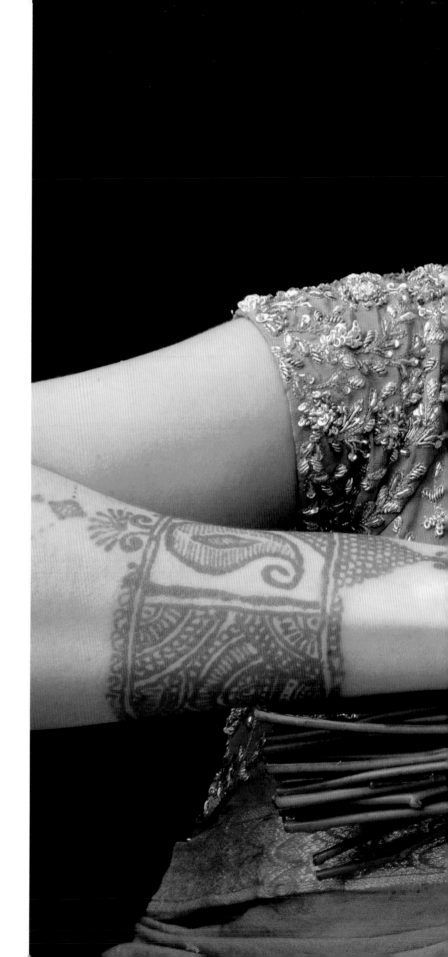

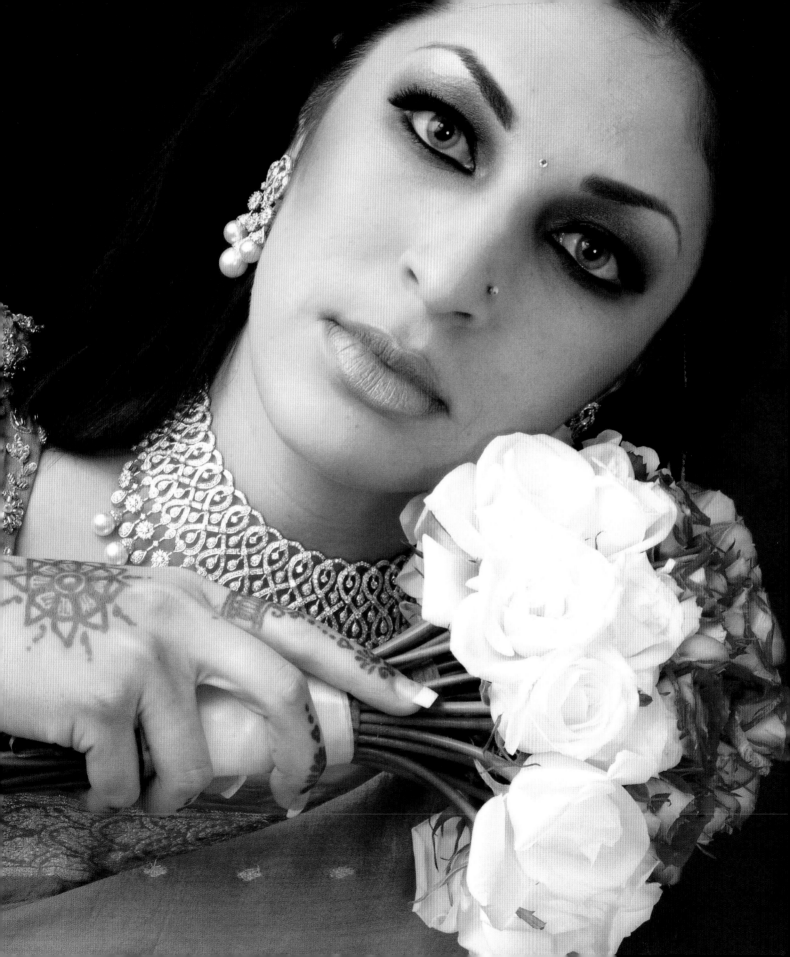

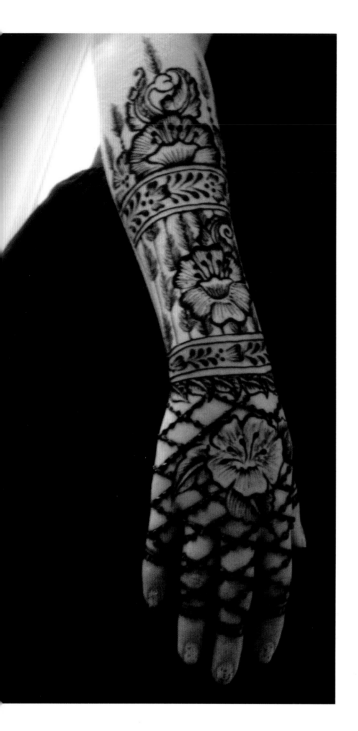

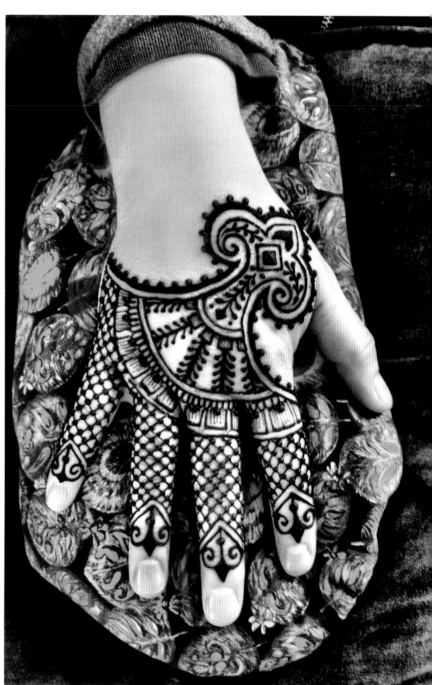

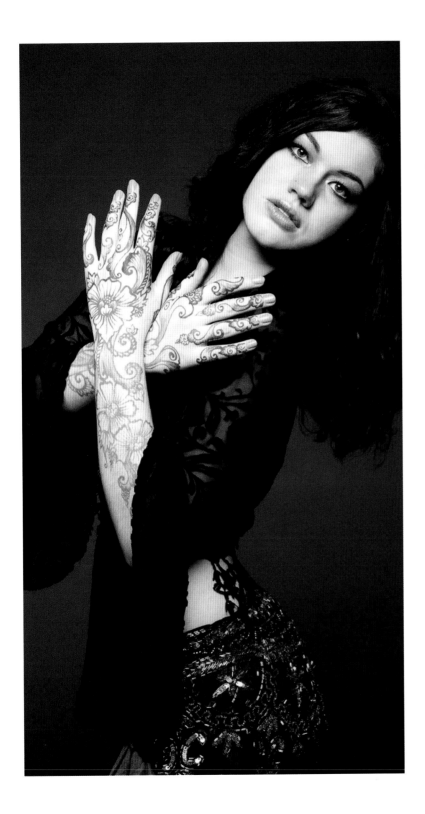

Genevieve Levin creates bold statement designs that are beautifully feminine yet strong and dynamic (opposite and left). She is also a multimedia artist who creates vibrant artwork with acrylic, paper, fabric, found objects, and all things that shine.

The belly and feet designs (overleaf) by Darcy Vasudev are clean, open and celebratory.

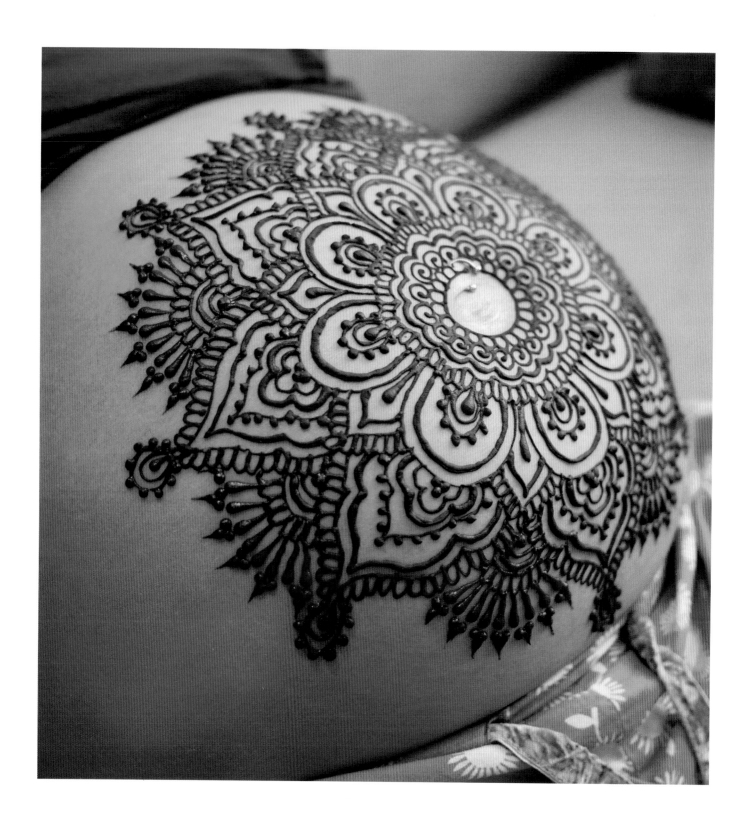

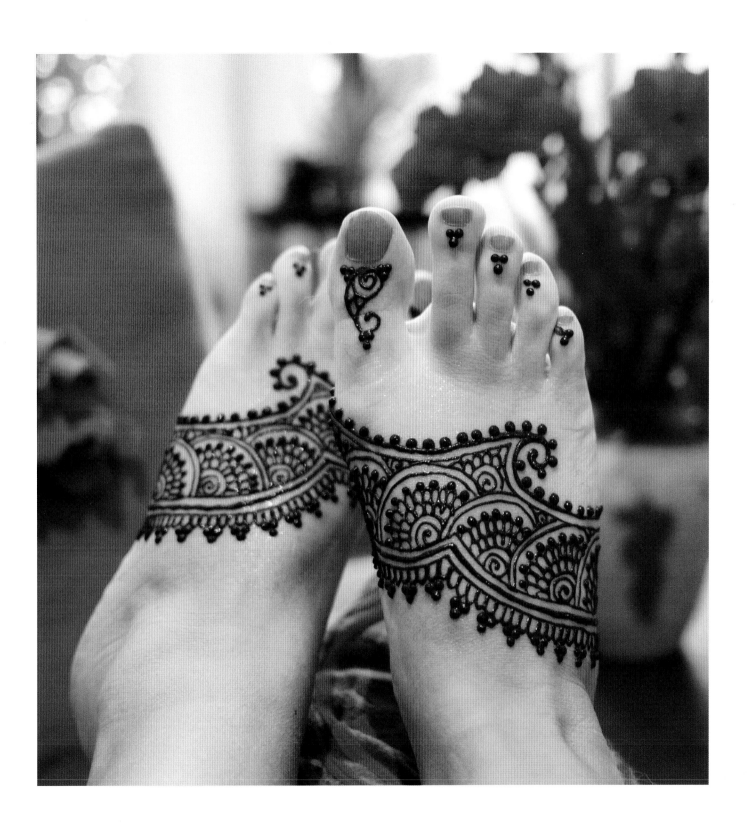

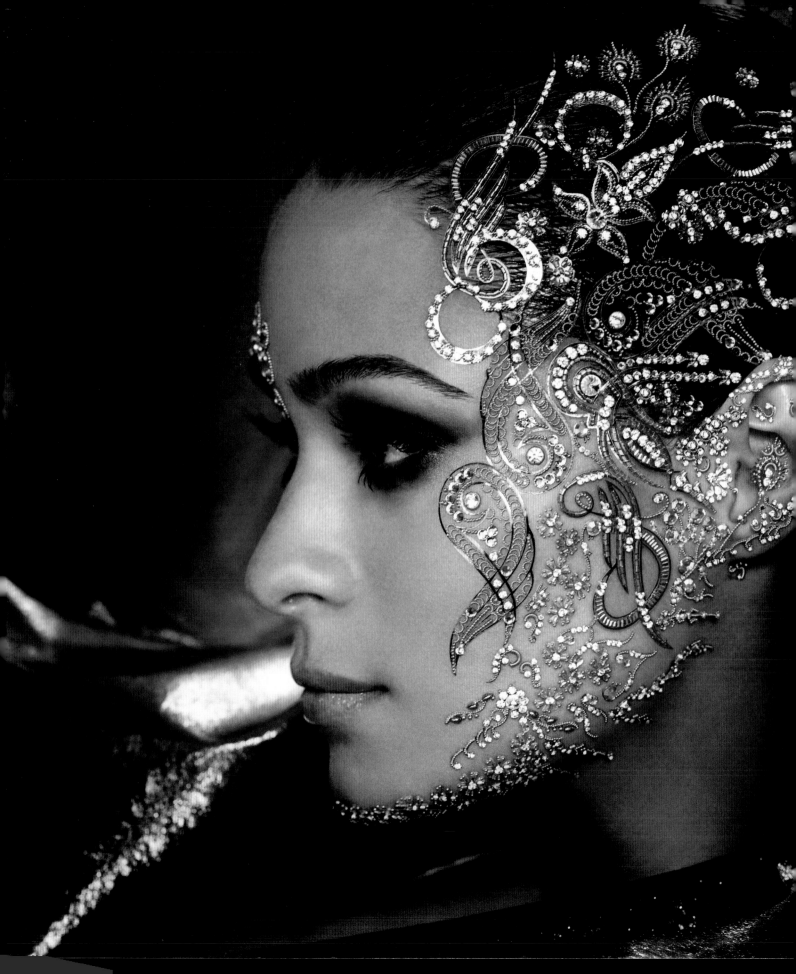

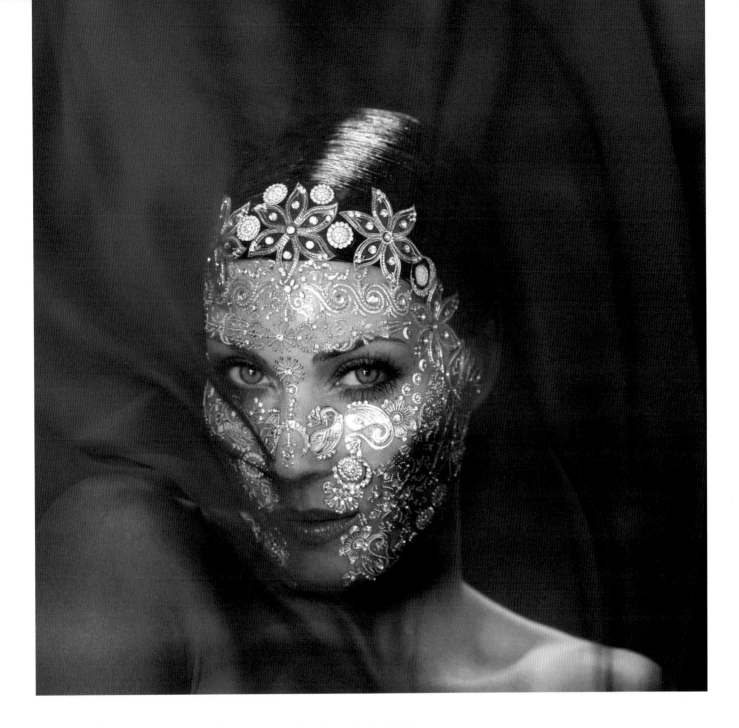

Once in a while a project and opportunity comes along that stays with you. I had the rare privilege to work alongside one of the best makeup artists in the world – Francesca Tolot. Her talented husband Alberto Tolot shot these photographs of her work (opposite and above). The images need no words, they speak and showcase the level and artistry of both individuals.

RESOURCES

ARTISTS

Genevieve Levin

www.remarkableblackbird.com
Making art has been a lifelong enterprise for southern Maine-based artist Genevieve Levin. A professional henna artist certified by the ICNHA (International Certification in Natural Henna Arts) since 2004, Nev is also a multimedia artist creating imaginative, vibrant artwork with acrylic, paper, fabric, found objects, and all things that shine. After earning her BFA from the Maine College of Art, Nev spent nine years working as a studio potter and art educator. In 2006, she made the decision to pursue her dream of running her own business and has since been a full-time henna artist. Her success with two businesses, ReMarkable Blackbird and Blackbird Studios, has been well worth the initial risk.

Her 'gypsy spirit' guides her to work in many situations: on the festival circuit, with other artists and belly dancers, belly blessings for mamas-to-be, brides on that big day and people undergoing treatment for cancer.

Credits include co-collaborating on the multi-award-winning short film *Unchastened*, features in the *The New York Times* and wedding blogs, the Intercontinental Hotel Diwali Celebration and the Maine Maritime Museum. Her images appear in books and magazines from New England to China and she is a featured presenter at numerous conferences throughout the year.

Her core belief about the world is that we are all connected through pattern, both visual and hidden, and she is passionate about maintaining that connection in her work with henna.

Prabhuti Patel

www.zibabeauty.com
The lead mehndi artist at Ziba Beauty, Prabhuti Patel has been on staff since 2006. Her creativity is only outshined by her beautiful smile and personality. She is not only detail-oriented, but a fast learner and her specialty is the art of glitter mehndi. Her attention to detail, patience and creativity outrank many other artists in this medium. She works out of the Ziba studio in Cerritos, California.

Kiran Sahib

www.kiransahib.com
An internationally recognized henna artist who is both highly creative and inspirationally unique, Kiran takes great pleasure in creating innovative and visually stunning henna designs for her clients. With over nine years of experience in the henna industry and a background in art, Kiran is seriously passionate about henna and it shows in her work. Known for her distinctive, clean, flowing and contemporary designs, she is heavily influenced by Indian and Arabic art. As well as cultural influence, her designs also incorporate images from nature, including flowers, leaves and birds.

Francesca Tolot

www.francescatolot.com
There's a reason that Francesca Tolot is known as one of the most skilled makeup artists in the business: it is her exquisite colour sensibility and the fine arts background that she brings to her craft. In today's environment, so-called celebrity makeup artists are a dime a dozen, but it's a precious few that have the impressive following of Hollywood greats, from the late Elizabeth Taylor to Catherine Zeta-Jones and Eva Longoria. In the music arena, Francesca's work with Beyoncé has received global recognition, namely on her stunning looks on her videos, red carpet events, and the *Dreamgirls* film. Finally, Francesca received great honours in accepting the First Annual Lucie Award for Makeup Artist of the Year.

Darcy Vasudev

www.hennalounge.com
A henna artist based in the San Francisco Bay Area, Darcy was born into an artistic family and began painting at the age of two. She first noticed henna in an old issue of *National Geographic* and, disappointed that the henna recipes were not described, began her own haphazard experiments. Introduced to Moroccan-style henna by a friend, Darcy soon began hennaing any friends or relatives that would sit still.

Since then, she has developed her own techniques and perfected her 'secret family recipe'. The search for a body-art-quality henna also led Darcy to begin importing fresh henna directly from Rajasthan, India. Now she has a full line of organic body art supplies and a sister business Henna Lounge Bazaar.

ABOUT ZIBA BEAUTY

Our family was the first to bring the ancient tradition of brow and body artistry to the West, beginning with Ziba Beauty and continuing the tradition with Sumita Beauty. At Sumita Beauty and Ziba Beauty we combine all our authentic experience to give you the very best experience and results. We define an entirely new level of service with our expertly trained beauty artists, our proprietary products and clean, modern, fashionable studios. We are setting a new standard, a new level of service and a different category of experience, bringing authentic Eastern beauty to the modern world.

Ziba Beauty is now franchising. Log onto zibafranchise.com for more information. To find a Ziba Beauty Studio near you log onto Zibabeauty.com.

WEBSITES AND SHOPS

UK

The Body Art Shop
www.bodyartshop.com
0161 408 3344
Powders, kits and cones.

Body Deco
www.bodydeco.co.uk
47 Station Road
Keswick, Cumbria CA12 4TW
017687 75812
Tattoos and transfers, stencils and kits plus a team of registered henna artists.

The Green Room
greenroomswirral.co.uk
6 Mill Lane
Wallasey, Wirral CH44 5UG
0151 200 9588
Professionally trained mehndi artists.

Henna Garden
www.henna-garden.co.uk
13 Creed Court
Westfield Way
London E1 4NS
Powder, glitter, kits and paints, as well as training courses are on offer.

Hennacat
hennacat.com
Carefully sourced henna products for hair and mehndi body art.

Simply Glitter
www.simplyglitter.co.uk
79 College Road
Harrow, Middlesex HA1 1BD
Kits, glitter, body art supplies, crystals, stencils and instructional videos.

USA

The Body Arts Company
www.bodyarts.com
800 300 9901
Quality products, including henna, body paint and books as well as a list of artists available for commission.

Earthues
www.earthues.com
5129 Ballard Ave NW
Seattle, WA 98107
206 789 1065
Fresh henna, products and kits.

Earth Henna
www.earthhenna.com
Lakaye Studio
6025 Santa Monica Blvd
Suite 202
Los Angeles, CA 90038
323 460 7333
Kits, stencils and books.

Henna and Henna Products
www.hennasupply.com
Marketplace for specific products, suppliers and trade.

Henna Lounge Bazaar
www.hennaloungebazaar.com
415 800 4800
Henna products and supplies, including powder, glitter, pre-filled cones and books.

Henna USA
www.hennausa.com
888 659 9595
516 808 8973
Suppliers of henna paste, powder, cones, books and kits.

Little India Stores
www.littleindianewyork.com
128 East 28th Street
New York, NY 10016
212 683 1691
Suppliers of henna powder and kits.

Ziba Beauty Center
www.zibabeauty.com
17832 Pioneer Blvd.
Artesia, CA 90701
562 402 5131
Kits, products and commissions available. See the website for studio locations near you.

INDEX

PICTURE CREDITS

All illustrations are copyright © Sumita Batra, apart from those on pages 70–9, which are copyright © Kiran Sahib.

The publishers would like to thank the following sources for their kind permission to reproduce the pictures in this book:

Alamy: /Sue Wilson: 30

Camera Press/Barry J Holmes 40

Corbis/Bernard and Catherine Desjeux 31

James Davies Travel 22t, 22b, 24r

Lorraine Day 2, 6, 8, 4–53

et archive 12

Eye Ubiquitous/David Cumming 16l

Getty Images: /Steve Granitz: 33l, 38, /Jon Kopaloff: 33c,

Robert Harding Picture Library 15b, 20r

Image Bank 13, 24tl, 25

London Features International Ltd 39r

Niall McInerney 41

Magnum/Denis Stock 21

PA News 37

Rex Features Ltd 36l, /BDG 33r

Herb Ritts/Visages 35

Tony Stone Images 14, 15t, 16r, 17, 20l, 29l

Trip 27/H Rogers 28, 29r

Yogi Patel/Global Photography 16r, 44–5, 47, 54, 81–3, 88–91, 103, 104, 126–7, 130–3

As seen in *You and Your Wedding*
Photography by Iain Philpott 42r, 42l, 43

Every effort has been made to acknowledge correctly and contact the source and copyright holder of each picture.
   Carlton Books Limited apologizes for any unintentional errors or omissions which will be corrected in future editions of this book.

AUTHOR'S ACKNOWLEDGEMENTS

A project of this magnitude could not happen without the help of numerous special people whom I would like to thank with all my heart. At Ziba Beauty we give every client a Shukar card as part of their visit with us. 'Shukar' means gratitude in Hindi and one of my favourite quotes on gratitude is: 'Feeling gratitude and not expressing it is like wrapping a present and not giving it'.

First and foremost, I would like to thank my husband Jagdeep and my three beautiful children Maya, Kavan and Hansa. I am eternally grateful to you for your never-ending support, my dear husband and my babies. Papa and my sister Suman – you are my pillars and the wind beneath my wings. Thank you for always being there for me. I don't say it enough, I love you both dearly. Sanjay, you are not only my little brother but like a son to me. I am hoping to be reading your book one day soon. Jasvir, Soina, Jagmohan, Mumji and Papaji , Preeti and especially Bhavin – thank you for always being there. Tejpal – I miss and love you. I will always see you in rainbows.

My friends Ravi, Fehmida, Ritu, Anupa, Gauri – you each know how I feel about you, and your feedback and support have always been a source of strength for me. Peter Savick, Madeline Leonard and the Cloutier Remix team, thank you for your support and all the opportunities you have always sent my way. Navneet Chugh, thank you for all your support throughout the years. I really appreciate it.

This second edition would not have happened without the support of Lisa Dyer and the team at Carlton Books. Thank you for believing in me and my project. Tonya, Aaron, Meenu, Bobby, Kristina, Jordan and Oscar – your contributions to the book, my life and to Ziba are truly appreciated and will never be forgotten – thank you.

The artists who helped make this book more creative are friends and family to me. Prabhuti Patel, you are my right-hand henna artist and I cannot believe how far you have come. Phenomenal artistry! Kiran Sahib, it has been a pleasure to work with you and I hope to, one day, support your own book on mehndi. I would buy it! Reema, you are my little sister and a very talented artist. Don't ever stop painting. I would also like to thank Liz Wilde for all her hard work writing for the first edition. I would also like to thank all the artists – especially Francesca and Alberto Tolot for their contributions to the book.

Lucky and Sonia, thank you for opening your home in London for me always. Love you. George Hammer and Tracey Woodward – I cannot express my gratitude enough for trusting me and my brands. I look forward to our continued work together. Karen Berman thank you for all your help and support. I feel blessed to have all of you in my life.

Madonna, I will be eternally grateful to you. You have changed my life in ways that you will never know. Loretta Roome, your wisdom, insight and vision are some of the reasons for mehndi's worldwide introduction. I will always remain proud of your accomplishments.

I have always been seen in the forefront, but the people who make me what I am are my supporting family and friend. If I have forgotten anyone, please forgive me.Lastly and most importantly, I would like to dedicate this book to my mom, without whom I would be nothing. Mom – I am everything I am – because you loved and believed in me. Shukria!